i

Nourished to Thrive

A Cancer Thriver's Food Memoir

By Dr. Diana C. Awuor

Dedication

To my husband, Sgt. Kennedy O. Osara, and our daughters Kendi Jeanne, Keana Anaya, and Kenna Arella your love, strength, and laughter gave me reason to persist and thrive.

To my mother, Mary Collete, and my sister, Olivia Benta, thank you for nourishing me with love and care through the most difficult season of my life. Your hands prepared my meals, your hearts carried my pain, and your presence gave me strength through every moment of my bilateral mastectomy and chemotherapy. I am here because you stood beside me with unwavering devotion and grace.

Author's Note

This book is my diet memoir. It is the story of how I walked through diagnosis, surgery, chemotherapy, and recovery, and how nutrition became one of my greatest allies. The meals, recipes, and reflections here were created in consultation with oncology dieticians and nutritionists at MD Anderson Cancer Centre - tailored to the diagnosis I received, the treatment I went through, and my healing journey. This book is not a prescription. It is not a substitute for professional medical advice. It is my story, what I did, what helped me, and what I still do to this day. If you are a patient, thriver, caregiver, or someone simply seeking clean eating for health, I hope you will find encouragement here. But always consult your own medical team before making changes to your diet or treatment plan. I prefer to call myself a thriver rather than a 'survivor,' because thriving is active and forward-looking. Still, this book is also useful for those who prefer the term 'survivor,' since hospitals and systems often use it.

Foreword

Having journeyed with Dr. Diana Awuor through her treatment and since our early years in elementary school, I have been privileged to witness her unwavering faith, discipline, and commitment to holistic healing. As both her long-time friend and a Biochemist and Food Scientist, I was honored to walk beside her, translating complex nutritional recommendations from her oncology dietitians into practical, culturally relevant strategies. My involvement often entailed integrating Kenyan traditional foods into her prescribed diet, ensuring accurate portioning, nutrient balance, and alignment with her therapeutic goals.

Our professional collaboration extended beyond her personal recovery. Together, we have served within the International Pleroma Convocation (IPC) Africa, an organization dedicated to supporting cancer patients undergoing infusion chemotherapy. Through IPC, we developed weekly meal plans designed to meet the nutritional needs of patients while respecting their cultural preferences and local food systems. This experience reaffirmed the vital role that nutrition plays, not only in sustaining life but also in restoring it.

Nourished to Thrive stands as both a testimony and a scientific contribution. It bridges the divide between research and real-world application, presenting nutrition as an integral component of cancer management. The book offers valuable insights for patients, survivors, caregivers, and healthcare professionals, emphasizing the intricate relationship between food, healing, and resilience.

Drawing from empirical evidence and lived experience, Dr. Diana Awuor exemplifies how science and personal narrative can merge to illuminate new pathways toward wellness. Her work reinforces a timeless principle that food, when thoughtfully chosen and prepared, can serve as medicine.

Jane Maurine Gati, *PhD. Biochemistry Candidate*

Biochemist, Educator, and Cancer Nutrition Advocate

Preface

For years, people asked me about the foods I eat, the recipes I use, and the nutritional plans that carried me through treatment. I am not a nutritionist; I am someone who received a cancer diagnosis and walked a long road of healing. Writing this book allows me to share, openly and practically, the nutrition framework that helped me thrive. I share this so that patients, thrivers, caregivers, and clean eaters everywhere have something solid to refer to, a guide rooted in lived experience, and supported by medical wisdom.

Table of Contents

PART ONE

Nutrition During Chemotherapy

During chemotherapy, I followed a structured plan created with my oncology dieticians at MD Anderson: three main meals, two snacks, and a small midnight protein shake to protect my gut overnight. Portions were tailored to my BMI and protein needs. Below was my exact daily rhythm and a 7-day plan with portions.

My Daily Structure

Half an hour before workout, I drank warm water mixed with fresh lemon juice. I took my breakfast after working out. My breakfast was mostly freshly juiced vegetable juice and vegan protein powder (single-ingredient: pea, mung bean, or chickpea). I tried to avoid fruit-only juices and add psyllium husk often to complement my fiber intake, as needed. When my appetite allowed, I replaced protein powder with boiled legumes such as mung beans, lentils, peas, or egg whites often alternating between them. Whether I managed to take the vegetable juice in the morning or not, I always made sure to drink it at some point during the day. That was a must-have, and it still is. I remember one of my doctors, who was also a cancer thriver, telling me after learning about the diagnosis, "Make sure you eat two medium-sized carrots every day." Juicing made that possible. I often included beetroot or celery in the mix.

My lunches and dinners comprised of leafy greens and plant protein or fish/hard organic chicken as advised by my team; portions listed below. I ate nutrient-dense and gentle options of snacks between meals to avoid long gaps. Lastly, when a chemotherapy nurse told me to protect my stomach lining from the corrosion of chemotherapy by drinking a midnight protein shake, I never stopped doing that until I completed my chemotherapy treatment. To prepare this shake, I mixed almond milk and a vegan protein powder. I wish I had started this sooner. I only learned about it late from the nurse, but even then, I decided to begin anyway despite chemotherapy having already damaged my gut and leaving me with IBS. Thankfully, I can confidently say it isn't a severe case of IBS; it was salvaged to some extent.

The Importance of Protein

Protein determined whether I could continue treatment on time. At the point of my diagnosis, I had decided to go fully vegan. I was convinced that meat had played a role in what had happened to me. I had been a heavy beef eater, fried chicken, oily takeouts, the kind of junk food I once called comfort. So, when my doctors suggested I include healthy animal protein like salmon or free-range organic chicken, I refused. I felt I was doing the right thing for my body, cleansing it of all the things that I believed had led me there. But what I didn't understand then was how my body worked differently. I knew I carried the sickle cell gene from my late father, but I didn't know how that could complicate treatment. My blood levels were already lower than average because of the trait, meaning my body needed good, consistent protein to maintain healthy blood production. The moment I received my first dose of carboplatin for the triple-negative tumor, my blood counts dropped sharply. My hemoglobin, white blood cells, everything fell too low for the next chemotherapy. The treatment had to be delayed. I wasn't too alarmed at first; I thought I could fix it with food my kind of food. I soaked and boiled lentils, made thick bean stews, ate peas, all believing that would raise my counts. But the more I tried, the worse it got. Then came the second cancellation. My medical oncologist looked at me kindly but firmly: "If you miss chemotherapy a third time, the treatment may not be effective." That day, as my family and close friends gathered with me on a Zoom call, the silence was heavy. Some were crying quietly, others trying to be strong. And then my dear friend, Mercy Kasuku, spoke up with a voice that shook but carried authority: "Diana, stop thinking only of yourself. Think of your children." Those words pierced my heart. I realized that I was trying to heal my way, not the way that could actually save me. That day, I humbled myself and said to my mom (she was also on the Zoom call), "Please prepare omena. I'll eat when I get home." Within two weeks of adding omena and salmon to my meals, my blood counts rose so beautifully that my doctor smiled and said, "This doesn't look like it belongs to a cancer patient." It was a turning point for me, a moment of surrender and revelation. I learned that food is not just about belief; it's about understanding the science of your body. From that moment on, I followed my team's guidance faithfully. I learned to balance faith with wisdom, conviction with knowledge. Every plate became a symbol of partnership between what I believed and what my body truly needed to heal.

My 7-Day Chemotherapy Meal Plan

Table 1.1: Monday Meal Plan

Time/Meal	Menu	Notes
Pre-workout	Warm water + lemon	30 min before workout
Breakfast	Green juice (cucumber, kale/spinach, celery, lemon, ginger) + vegan protein	Blend protein into juice; add 1 tsp psyllium if needed
Snack 1	Soaked almonds or chia pudding (almond milk)	Gentle on digestion
Lunch	Leafy salad + protein (Option A: lentils; Option B: 120 g salmon/omena)	Add cucumber, tomatoes; dress with citrus/herb dressing
Snack 2	Almond yogurt + berries	Probiotic support
Dinner	Red-lentil Turmeric Soup + Steamed Greens and Vegetable Juice (Carrots, Ginger and Celery Juice)	Warm, easy to digest; no oil
Midnight shake	Vegan Protein Shake (almond milk)	Protect gut overnight (IBS)

Juicing Notes

Base: cucumber, kale/spinach, celery, lemon, ginger. Portion: 350–400 ml per serving. Blend the juice with vegan protein powder to support muscle repair and stable blood sugar.

Table 1:2: My Tuesday Meal Plan

Time/Meal	Menu	Notes
Pre-workout	Warm water + lemon	
Breakfast	Green juice + Vegan protein (add kiwi or green apple skin)	Add fiber from skin
Snack 1	Carrot + Cucumber Sticks with Hummus	Oil-free hummus
Lunch	Zucchini "pasta" with Cherry Tomato Basil Sauce + Hemp "parmesan"	Low-carb, high fiber
Snack 2	Almond yogurt + Chia Seeds	Omega-3 from Chia
Dinner	White Bean + Spinach Soup	Soft texture; no garlic
Midnight shake	Vegan Protein Shake and Vegetable Juice (Carrots, Ginger and Beetroot Juice)	

From My Diary: The Beetroot Scare

One day, when I went to the restroom, I froze. The color in the toilet bowl was red not faintly pink, but a deep, frightening red. My heart started pounding. My mind immediately went to the worst possible place. Had the cancer spread? Was I bleeding internally? Was this the end starting to unfold? Panic gripped me. I called my mother. She had travelled from Kenya to the United States to take care of me and the kids during my chemotherapy. My sister, Olivia, had been with me during surgery and through my healing afterward. I could barely speak through tears. "Mom," I cried, "something is wrong! There's blood in my stool." She listened quietly. My mother is a retired nurse but I was a stubborn patient. I only trusted my medical oncologist. You see, my mom, being a pastor as well, had earlier told me there was no need for chemotherapy because she believed I was already healed. I told her not to say that again, that I was going to complete the full treatment.

I know my mom, having practiced as a nurse, was also scared because she understood what chemotherapy could do. She consoled me, told me everything would be fine, and then prayed for me. Still shaken, I contacted my oncologist immediately. She scheduled an appointment for blood work the same day, followed by a consultation to discuss the findings. The results showed nothing alarming. Then she asked me what I had been eating. I told her everything the vegetables, the juice, and finally mentioned the beetroot. My mom was on speakerphone during the appointment. When the doctor smiled and said, "Yes, beetroot can turn your stool and even urine reddish. It's harmless just pigments passing through your system," I felt both embarrassed and relieved. Then my mom laughed and said, "I knew it was the beetroot, but since you only believe Dr. O on treatment matters, I didn't want to tell you." We all laughed together me, my mom, and my doctor. That moment taught me a lesson I will never forget: healing is not just about medicine; it's about awareness. It's about understanding what natural foods can do the colors, the smells, the reactions so that we don't let fear control our minds. The Beetroot Scare became one of those stories that I laugh about now, but at that time, it reminded me how deeply cancer can train your mind to anticipate the worst. It was a lesson in humility, knowledge, and calm to always observe before panicking, and to trust that sometimes, nature is just painting its own colors inside you.

Table 1.3: My Wednesday Meal Plan

Time/Meal	Menu	Notes
Pre-workout	Warm Water + Lemon	
Breakfast	Green Juice + Vegan Protein	
Snack 1	Almonds + Blueberries	
Lunch	Spinach Salad + Lentil Patties (Baked, Oil-Free)	See recipe
Snack 2	Hummus + Cucumber	
Dinner	Eggplant Rollatini (Cashew Cheese) + Steamed Kale and Vegetable Juice (Carrots and Celery)	Baked covered; no char
Midnight Shake	Vegan Protein Shake	

Table 1.4: My Thursday Meal Plan

Time/Meal	Menu	Notes
Pre-workout	Warm Water + Lemon	
Breakfast	Green Juice + Vegan Protein	
Snack 1	Chia Pudding with Almond Milk	
Lunch	Salad + Salmon	
Snack 2	Almond Yogurt + Kiwi	
Dinner	Red-Lentil Turmeric Soup + Steamed Broccoli and Vegetable Juice (Carrots and Beetroot)	Limit crucifers if too gassy
Midnight shake	Vegan Protein Shake	

Table 1.5: My Friday Meal Plan

Time/Meal	Menu	Notes
Pre-workout	Warm Water + Lemon	
Breakfast	Green Juice + Vegan Protein (Add Celery)	
Snack 1	Cucumber + Carrot Sticks with Hummus	
Lunch	Portobello "Steak" + Cauliflower Mash + Greens (Steamed Spinach)	Steam-sauté; rice vinegar marinade
Snack 2	Almond Yogurt + Berries	
Dinner	Lentil Curry (Yellow/Red) + Spinach and Vegetable Juice (Carrots and Celery)	Mild spices; no garlic
Midnight shake	Vegan Protein Shake	

Table 1.6: My Saturday Meal Plan

Time/Meal	Menu	Notes
Pre-workout	Warm Water + Lemon	
Breakfast	Protein Pancakes (Red Lentil or Chickpea) + Berries	Oil-free; see recipe
Snack 1	Soaked Almonds	
Lunch	Chickpea Salad Bowl (Greens, Cucumber, Tomato, Herbs)	Citrus/herb dressing
Snack 2	Almond Yogurt + Chia	
Dinner	Zucchini "Pasta" + Tomato Basil Sauce and Vegetable Juice (Carrots and Beetroot)	
Midnight shake	Vegan Protein Shake	

Table 1.7: My Sunday Meal Plan

Time/Meal	Menu	Notes
Pre-workout	Warm Water + Lemon	
Breakfast	Green Juice + Vegan Protein	Mix leafy vegetables and cruciferous vegetables. Different colors
Snack 1	Hummus + Veg Sticks	
Lunch	Spinach Salad + Lentils or Salmon/Omena	
Snack 2	Almond Yogurt + Berries	
Dinner	White Bean–Spinach Soup and Vegetable Juice (Carrots and Celery)	
Midnight shake	Vegan Protein Shake	

From My Diary: Importance of Community (Chemo-Day Rhythm)

Because of COVID-19 restrictions, I couldn't bring anyone with me into the chemo room. But I refused to go through it alone. So, I brought my people in through Zoom. Every chemo day had a rhythm. I informed my family and close friends via a WhatsApp group that had been created to journey with me. By the time the nurse connected the IV line, they were already there with me smiling, praying, laughing, encouraging. My community joined from Kenya, from across the U.S., and from wherever love could reach. We opened with prayer. Sometimes we sang softly, played music. Someone shared a verse or a word of encouragement. Even when fatigue hit, they stayed with me, cameras still on, letting me rest while their presence filled the room from miles away. The infusion was never lonely; it was a rhythm of faith surrounded by love. One nurse came over one time to inform me that another patient had complained about noise from my cubicle. Once she passed that messaged, she leaned closer and whispered, "Please keep doing what you're doing. It encourages the nurses." I smiled, deeply touched. In that sterile room, something holy was happening. My healing space had become a sanctuary where faith, friendship, and medicine met. Those sessions carried me through. What was supposed to be six long hours often felt like thirty minutes. My community didn't just show up; they carried me.

They made me laugh when I felt weak and prayed when I couldn't find words. Even across time zones and oceans, they reminded me that healing is not meant to be a solo journey. On May 15, 2021, I rang the bell at MD Anderson as my children watched on Zoom. Their faces glowed with joy as I read aloud the words every patient recites: "Ring this bell Three times well Its toll to clearly say, my treatment's done This course is run And I am on my way!" Tears rolled down my cheeks as I rang it, not just for myself but for everyone who had been part of that journey the doctors, nurses, friends, family, and all those who had prayed through the screen. That day reminded me how technology, often seen as a barrier, can also be a bridge. It can connect hearts across oceans, bring warmth into hospital rooms, and make presence possible even when distance won't allow physical touch. My community proved that love can travel through screens and still feel just as real.

My Common Recipes During Chemotherapy

Almond Milk (Homemade)

Ingredients:

- 1 cup raw almonds, soaked 8–12 hrs.
- 4 cups water
- Pinch Himalayan salt

Steps:

1. Drain and rinse-soaked almonds.
2. Blend with 4 cups water and a pinch of salt for 60–90 seconds.
3. Strain through a nut-milk bag. Yields ~4 cups. Refrigerate up to 3 days.

Almond Yogurt (No Oil)

Ingredients:

- 4 cups homemade almond milk
- 1 probiotic capsule (dairy-free)
- Pinch Himalayan salt

Steps:

1. Warm almond milk gently to lukewarm (not hot).
2. Open probiotic capsule; whisk contents into milk with a pinch of salt.
3. Pour into a clean jar, cover loosely, and ferment 10–12 hours in a warm place until tangy.
4. Refrigerate to set. Stir before serving.

Oil-Free Hummus (No Garlic)

Ingredients:

- 1½ cups cooked chickpeas (drained, reserve aquafaba)
- 3–4 Tbsp aquafaba (as needed)
- 3 Tbsp lemon juice
- 1 tsp cumin
- Pinch Himalayan salt

Steps:

1. Blend chickpeas with lemon juice, cumin, and 3 Tbsp aquafaba until smooth.
2. Add more aquafaba 1 Tbsp at a time for desired creaminess.
3. Season to taste.

Notes: Serve with cucumber and carrot sticks.

Red Lentil Turmeric Soup

Ingredients:

- 1 cup dry red lentils, rinsed
- 5 cups water/vegetable broth
- 1 tsp ground turmeric
- ½ tsp ground ginger
- ½ small onion, finely chopped (optional)
- Pinch Himalayan salt
- Black pepper to taste

Steps:

1. Combine lentils and water/broth in a pot; bring to a boil.
2. Add turmeric, ginger, onion (if using), and salt.
3. Reduce heat; simmer 15–18 minutes until creamy.
4. Season with black pepper. Serve with steamed greens.

Zucchini "Pasta" with Tomato Basil Sauce

Ingredients:

- 2 medium zucchini spiralized
- 1½ cups cherry tomatoes, halved
- ¼ small onion, minced (optional)
- 2 Tbsp chopped fresh basil
- 1–2 tsp rice vinegar
- Pinch Himalayan salt

Steps:

1. Steam-sauté onion (if using) with a splash of water until soft.

2. Add cherry tomatoes; simmer 6–8 minutes until saucy. Stir in basil, rice vinegar, and salt.

3. Lightly steam zucchini strands 1–2 minutes to soften (avoid overcooking).

4. Toss with sauce. Top with 2 Tbsp hemp seeds for protein.

Eggplant Rollatini (Cashew Cheese, Oil-Free)

Ingredients:

- 1 medium eggplant, sliced lengthwise ¼-inch
- 1 cup raw cashews, soaked 4 hrs.
- 2–3 Tbsp lemon juice
- ¼ cup water (as needed)
- 1 Tbsp chopped herbs (basil/parsley)
- Pinch Himalayan salt

Steps:

1. Blend cashews, lemon juice, salt, and just enough water into a thick cashew cheese. Stir in herbs.

2. Steam eggplant slices 3–4 minutes until pliable (or bake covered at 350°F/175°C 10–12 minutes; avoid charring).

3. Spread 1–2 Tbsp cashew cheese on each slice; roll and place in a baking dish.

4. Cover and bake 12–15 minutes at 350°F/175°C until warmed through.

Portobello "Steak" + Cauliflower Mash (Oil-Free)

Ingredients:

- 1 large portobello cap, cleaned
- 2 tsp rice vinegar
- 1 tsp lemon juice
- ½ tsp smoked paprika (optional)
- 2 cups cauliflower florets
- Pinch Himalayan salt

Steps:

1. Whisk rice vinegar, lemon juice, paprika, and salt; brush on mushroom.

2. Steam-sauté mushroom in a skillet with a splash of water 3–4 minutes per side; avoid charring.

3. Steam cauliflower until tender; mash with a splash of almond milk and salt.

Protein Pancakes (Red Lentil)

Ingredients:

- 1 cup red lentils, soaked 2–3 hrs. and drained
- ¾–1 cup water
- ½ tsp cumin
- Pinch Himalayan salt

Steps:

1. Blend-soaked lentils with ¾ cup water, cumin, and salt until smooth (add up to 1 cup water for pourable batter).

2. Cook on a non-stick pan over medium heat, 2–3 minutes per side, without oil.

Notes: Serve with ½ cup berries.

Protein Pancakes (Chickpea)

Ingredients:

- 1 cup chickpea flour (besan)
- 1¼ cups water
- Pinch Himalayan salt
- 1 Tbsp chopped herbs (optional)

Steps:

1. Whisk chickpea flour, water, salt, and herbs until smooth; rest 15–20 minutes.

2. Cook on a non-stick pan over medium heat, 2–3 minutes per side, without oil.

PART TWO

The Routine that Sustains my Healing

Nutrition after Treatment

After treatment, I continued with the same meal plan for several months in fact, for almost a year before my diet began to change. As my body healed, my hair started growing back, the new nails coming in were no longer dark, and my complexion began to return. Naturally, my meal plan evolved with my recovery. I no longer needed to eat five times a day; as my schedule shifted, I returned to three balanced meals. Finding a routine that worked for me, however, was not easy. I no longer had help it was just my husband and me again, managing everything with the kids. My meals were often different from theirs, which made things even more complicated. After many struggles trying to figure out what could fit both my healing journey and our family rhythm without leaving me drained, stressed, or exhausted from preparing separate meals I finally discovered a pattern that was both healthy and manageable. This routine has served me well, even now that I work full-time. I appreciate it because it changes each month, so I never get bored or feel stuck in one cycle for too long. Below, I share the plan that has continued to sustain me.

Food Portion Control

Please note that the meal plans in this guide do not include my personal portion measurements intentionally. Every person's body is unique, and I don't want anyone basing their food portions on mine. To make the most of these recipes, I encourage you to calculate your own Body Mass Index (BMI) and use it to guide your portion sizes. This helps you eat in a way that supports your body composition, energy needs, and wellness goals, whether your focus is maintaining, losing, or gaining healthy weight.

How to Calculate and Understand Your BMI

Your BMI can be calculated using this simple formula:

BMI = weight (kg) ÷ [height (m)] ^{2}

For example, if you weigh 70 kilograms and are 1.65 meters tall, your BMI would be: $70 ÷ (1.65 × 1.65) = 25.7$

Once you know your BMI, you can use it to understand your body's general nutritional needs:

- A BMI below 18.5 means you are underweight and may need slightly larger portions and more frequent, balanced meals.

- A BMI between 18.5 and 24.9 is considered healthy — you can maintain your current balance, focusing on clean, nutrient-dense foods.

- A BMI between 25 and 29.9 falls in the overweight range, where smaller portions and higher vegetable intake can support weight balance.

- A BMI of 30 or higher suggests that smaller, consistent portions and a focus on high-fiber, high-protein meals with plenty of hydration will be most beneficial.

How to Portion According to Your BMI

Use your BMI as a guide, not a restriction. The goal is to nourish your body in a balanced, sustainable way. You don't need to measure every meal — you can rely on simple visual cues:

- Protein (meat, legumes, or fish): About the size of your palm (1–2 servings depending on your BMI and activity level).

- Vegetables: Fill half your plate. These are rich in fiber and support digestion and hormone balance.

- Whole grains or starches: Roughly the size of your cupped hand or skip them for low-carb meals. I rarely include starches in my meals. When I do, I choose wholesome options such as quinoa, sweet potatoes, black rice, arrowroot, and pumpkin.

- Healthy fats: About a thumb-sized amount (from avocado, chia seeds, or soaked almonds).

- Smoothies: One tall glass (8–10 ounces) is a full serving.

If you are working with a nutritionist or healthcare provider, they can help you adjust your portions even more precisely based on your individual goals and health needs.

Breakfast Choices for a Well-Balanced Meal

My breakfasts are usually fresh vegetable juices blended with a scoop of protein powder. I prefer starting my day with something light, clean, and easy to fix, especially since I eat only two main meals a day. This approach keeps my mornings energized without feeling heavy.

That's also why you'll notice that my lunches are mostly salads and my dinners are smoothies simple, nutrient-dense, and quick to prepare.

However, you can adjust this routine to suit your needs. If you prefer a solid meal for breakfast instead of juicing, that's perfectly fine. The key is to ensure that each meal remains well balanced by following the portion control formula outlined earlier.

Healthy Breakfast Ideas
- Quinoa pancakes made with almond milk or yogurt

- Amaranth porridge topped with sliced berries or chia seeds

- Steamed vegetables with egg whites and avocado

- Smoothie bowl with blended kale, almond milk, and a spoonful of nut butter

- Scrambled egg whites with spinach and a side of lightly roasted sweet potato

- Overnight oats made with amaranth flakes, coconut yogurt, and cinnamon

- Vegetable omelet paired with a small serving of quinoa

Monthly Meal Plans After My Breast Cancer Treatment: January

This January plan reflects the structured healing nutrition I followed after chemotherapy. It contains exact ingredients, portions, and measurements for each meal, ensuring balance of protein, fiber, and anti-inflammatory foods.

Table 2.1: January - Monday

Meal	Menu	Notes
Breakfast	Juice: Carrots, Beetroot, Cucumber, Kale, Ginger, Lemon + Pea Protein	Add psyllium husk
Lunch	Spinach & Arugula Salad + Mung Beans, Cucumber, Cherry Tomatoes and Herbs	Orange juice dressing
Dinner	Smoothie: Almond Milk, Spinach, Blueberries and Chia. Side: Mixed Beans with Herbs and Lime (boiled until soft, tossed with chopped cilantro, onion, and a splash of lime juice).	Light, anti-inflammatory

Table 2.1: January - Tuesday

Meal	Menu	Notes
Breakfast	Juice: Carrot, Celery, Cucumber, Spinach, Kiwi, Ginger + Chickpea Protein	Fiber boost from kiwi
Lunch	Kale Salad + Salmon, Cucumber, Tomato, Steamed Broccoli	Steam or bake covered, no charring
Dinner	Smoothie: Steamed Spinach, Almond Milk, Strawberries, and avocado. Side: Green peas with mint and basil, steamed and mixed with finely shredded mint leaves and basil for a refreshing flavor.	Hormone balance support

Table 2.3: January - Wednesday

Meal	Menu	Notes
Breakfast	Juice: Carrots, Cucumber, Kale, Beetroot, Lemon, Ginger + Mung Bean Protein	Beet supports blood health
Lunch	Salad: Arugula Salad + Chickpeas, Avocado, Cucumber, Tomato, Herbs	Citrus dressing
Dinner	Smoothie: Almond Milk, Steamed Arugula, Cubed Carrots and Raspberries Side: Baked hard chicken (season with rosemary + cumin + crushed coriander seeds)	Antioxidant-rich

Table 2.4: January - Thursday

Meal	Menu	Notes
Breakfast	Juice: 2 Medium Sized Carrots, 1 Medium Sized Beetroot, 1 Small Cucumber, 1 Cup of Kale, ½ Green Apple Skin, 1-Inch Ginger + Chickpea Protein	Fiber from apple skin
Lunch	Salad: Spinach Salad + Air Fried Salmon, Cherry Tomatoes and Green Onions	Protein-dense; no oil frying
Dinner	Smoothie: Almond Milk, Mixed Greens, Red Bell Peppers, Blueberries and Avocado. Side: Lentils or beans (flavored with ginger + green onions+ parsley)	Anti-inflammatory blend

Table 2.5: January - Friday

Meal	Menu	Notes
Breakfast	Juice: Carrots, Celery, Cucumber, Spinach, Lemon (with peels) + Mung Bean Protein + Orange	Balanced breakfast I often add cinnamon, turmeric, black pepper and psyllium husk. The psyllium husk is to increase fiber
Lunch	Salad: Chopped Kale + Boiled Cannellini Beans, Boiled Lentils, Cucumber, Tomato and Bell Pepper	White beans for protein & fiber I use one of my dressings. Check my dressing recipes
Dinner	Smoothie: Almond Milk, Steamed Spinach, Cubed Carrots and Blackberries. Side: Baked wild salmon with herbs (flavored with ginger + thyme + lemon zest).	Gut-healing focus I don't use garlic because of irritable bowel syndrome (IBS). You can always add garlic to yours.

Table 2.6: January - Saturday

Meal	Menu	Notes
Breakfast	Juice: Carrots, Cucumber, Medium Beetroot, Kale, Kiwi, Ginger + Pea Protein	Vitamin C-rich juice You can replace cucumber with some water
Lunch	Salad: Spinach + Black-Eyed Peas, Cucumber, Tomato and Herbs	Protein-rich legumes
Dinner	Smoothie: Steamed Mixed Greens, Cubed Red Bell Peppers, Almond Milk, Raspberries and Hemp Seeds. Side: Chickpeas with cumin and lemon (boiled tender, then tossed with ground cumin, ginger, and fresh lemon juice)	Immune boost

Table 2.7: January - Sunday

Meal	Menu	Notes
Breakfast	Juice: Carrots, Celery, Cucumber, Kale, Lemon with Skin + Chickpea Protein Powder + Ginger	Fiber and detox support
Lunch	Boiled Omena, Steamed White Cabbage with Green Onions, Cherry Tomatoes and Millet Ugali	Iron-rich protein
Dinner	Smoothie: Steamed Spinach, Red Cabbage, Almond Milk, Blueberries and Chia Side: Mixed beans with herbs and lime (boiled until soft, tossed warm with celery, chopped cilantro, and a splash of lime juice).	Anti-inflammatory dinner

January Recap

January emphasizes clean resets with vegetable juices, high-protein legumes (mung beans, chickpeas, cannellini, black-eyed peas), salmon, omena, and hard organic chicken. Anti-inflammatory foods included turmeric, ginger, chia, hemp, berries, and leafy greens. Workouts (treadmill + light weights) complemented this plan, helping me restore strength and lower BMI.

Monthly Meal Plans After My Breast Cancer Treatment: February

This February plan continues the structured healing nutrition with full balance of proteins, fibers, and anti-inflammatory foods. Focus remains on leafy greens, beans, salmon, omena, and chicken.

Table 2.8: February - Monday

Meal	Menu	Notes
Breakfast	Juice: Carrots, Celery, Cucumber, Kale, Lemon + Ginger + Pea Protein	Add 1 tsp psyllium husk
Lunch	Spinach Salad + Boiled Lentils, Cucumber, Cherry Tomatoes, Herbs	Orange juice dressing
Dinner	Smoothie: Almond Milk, Spinach, Steamed Cauliflower, Green Apple Peels. Side: Omena with tomato, onion, and ginger + chickpeas with cumin and lemon	Light, anti-inflammatory

Table 2.9: February - Tuesday

Meal	Menu	Notes
Breakfast	Juice: Carrots, Beetroot, Cucumber, Chopped Kale, Kiwi, Ginger + Chickpea Protein	Fiber boost from kiwi
Lunch	Salad: Arugula + Salmon, Cherry Tomatoes, Green Onions and Green Onions Side:	Steam or bake covered, no charring
Dinner	Smoothie: Steamed Mixture of Red and White Cabbage, Almond Milk, Strawberries, Hemp seeds. Side: Mung beans with ginger and herbs (boiled or lightly sprouted, then mixed with grated ginger, coriander, and leek greens for gentle spice).	Hormone balance support

Table 2.10: February - Wednesday

Meal	Menu	Notes
Breakfast	Juice: Carrots, Cucumber, Kale, Beetroot, Lemon, Ginger + Mung Bean Protein	Beet supports blood health
Lunch	Salad: Spinach + Boiled Chickpeas, Cucumber, Cherry Tomatoes and Herbs	Citrus dressing
Dinner	Smoothie: Almond Yogurt, Raspberries, Mixed Leafy Vegetables. Side: Green peas with mint and basil (steamed and mixed with finely shredded mint and basil for a fresh, cooling side).	Antioxidant-rich

Table 2.11: February - Thursday

Meal	Menu	Notes
Breakfast	Juice: Carrots, Celery, Cucumber, Spinach, Green Apple Skin, Ginger + Chickpea Protein	Fiber from apple skin
Lunch	Salad: Chopped Kale + Organic Chicken, Cucumber and Cherry Tomato	Protein-dense; no oil frying
Dinner	Smoothie: Almond Milk, Chopped Arugula, Blueberries, Ripe Banana, Chia Seeds. Side: Black-eyed peas with ginger and cumin (boiled soft and tossed with ginger, cumin, and a sprinkle of parsley).	Anti-inflammatory blend

Table 2.12: February - Friday

Meal	Menu	Notes
Breakfast	Juice: Carrots, Beetroot, Cucumber, Chopped Spinach, Lemon + Ginger + Mung Bean Protein	Balanced breakfast
Lunch	Salad: Chopped Arugula + Cannellini Beans, Cucumber, Cherry Tomato, Bell Pepper and Avocado	White beans for protein & fiber
Dinner	Smoothie: Almond Milk, Steamed Mixed Leafy Greens and Blackberries. Side: Pigeon peas with basil and lime (boiled until tender, then brightened with basil and a squeeze of lime).	Gut-healing focus

Table 2.13: February - Saturday

Meal	Menu	Notes
Breakfast	Juice: Carrots, Celery, Cucumber, Chopped Kale, Kiwi, Ginger + Pea Protein + Hemp Protein	Vitamin C-rich juice
Lunch	Salad: Chopped Spinach + Boiled Black-Eyed Peas, Cucumber, Tomato and Herbs	Protein-rich legumes
Dinner	Smoothie: Almond Milk, Steamed Collard Greens, Raspberries and Hemp Seeds. Side: Lightly toasted omena with tomato, onion, and a touch of ginger (dry-toasted, then simmered gently with tomato, onion tops, and fresh ginger for a savory, calcium-rich side).	Immune boost

Table 2.14: February - Sunday

Meal	Menu	Notes
Breakfast	Juice: Carrots, Celery, Cucumber, Chopped Spinach, Lemon, Ginger + Chickpea Protein	Fiber and detox support
Lunch	Salad: Chopped Kale + Omena, Cucumber and Cherry Tomato	Iron-rich protein
Dinner	Smoothie: Coconut Cultured Milk, Blueberries, Chia, Side: Lentils with Turmeric and Parsley cooked with Asafetida, (celery, and turmeric; topped with chopped parsley).	Anti-inflammatory dinner

February Recap

February continued with a variety of legumes (lentils, chickpeas, cannellini, black-eyed peas), fish (salmon, omena), and chicken. Berries, chia/hemp, turmeric, and leafy greens supported anti-inflammatory balance and healing.

Monthly Meal Plans After My Breast Cancer Treatment: March

This March plan continued to build strength and energy, emphasizing protein for muscle recovery and high fiber for gut health. By this time, treadmill walks (1 mile daily) and minimal weights were part of my rhythm. Protein intake after workouts was key in preventing muscle mass loss.

Table 2.15: March - Monday

Meal	Menu	Notes
Breakfast	Juice: Carrots, Celery, Cucumber, Kale, Lemon + Pea Protein	Add Psyllium Husk
Lunch	Salad: Arugula + Boiled Lentils, Green Onions, Cherry Tomato and Herbs	Citrus Dressing
Dinner	Smoothie: Almond Milk, Spinach, Blueberries and Chia Side: Black-Eyed Peas with Ginger and Cumin (Boiled Soft and Tossed with Ginger, Cumin, and a Sprinkle of Parsley).	Anti-Inflammatory

Table 2.16: March - Tuesday

Meal	Menu	Notes
Breakfast	Juice: Celery, Cucumber, Spinach, Kiwi, Ginger + Chickpea Protein	Kiwi for vitamin C
Lunch	Salad: Spinach + Air fried Salmon, Tomato, Mixed Greens	Steam or Bake Covered, No Charring
Dinner	Smoothie: Almond Milk, Strawberries and Hemp Seeds Side: Cannellini Beans with Celery and Lemon (Boiled Until Creamy, Finished with Celery, Thyme, and Lemon Zest).	Supports Hormone Balance

Table 2.17: March - Wednesday

Meal	Menu	Notes
Breakfast	Juice: Carrots, Cucumber, Kale, Beetroot, Lemon, Ginger + Mung Bean Protein	Beet Supports Blood Levels
Lunch	Salad: Red Cabbage + Chickpeas, Avocado, Cucumber, Cherry Tomato and Herbs	Healthy Fats & Fiber
Dinner	Smoothie: Almond Milk, Raspberries and Chia Side: Baked Wild Salmon with Herbs + Red Lentils with Ginger and Celery.	Antioxidant-Rich

Table 2.18: March - Thursday

Meal	Menu	Notes
Breakfast	Juice: Celery, Cucumber, Kale, Green Apple Skin, Ginger + Chickpea Protein	Fiber From Apple Skin
Lunch	Salad: Spinach + Hard Organic Chicken, Cucumber, Cherry Tomatoes and Carrots	Protein Dense; No Oil Frying
Dinner	Smoothie: Almond Milk, Blueberries and Hemp Side: Mixed beans with herbs and lime (kidney, black, and white beans boiled soft, tossed with celery, cilantro, and lime juice).	Anti-Inflammatory Blend

Table 2.19: March - Friday

Meal	Menu	Notes
Breakfast	Juice: Carrots, Celery, Cucumber, Spinach, Lemon + Mung Bean Protein	Balanced Breakfast
Lunch	Salad: Arugula + Cannellini Beans, Cucumber, Green Onions, Cherry Tomato and Bell Pepper	Cannellini Beans for Protein & Fiber
Dinner	Smoothie: Almond Milk, Blackberries and Chia Side: Lightly Toasted Omena with Tomato, Onion, and a Touch of Ginger (Dry-Toasted, then Simmered Gently with Tomato, Onion and Fresh Ginger for a Savory, Calcium-Rich Side).	Gut-Healing Focus

Table 2.20: March - Saturday

Meal	Menu	Notes
Breakfast	Juice: Carrots, Cucumber, Kale, Kiwi, Ginger + Pea Protein	Vitamin C-Rich Juice
Lunch	Salad: Spinach + Black-Eyed Peas, Cucumber, Tomato and Herbs	Protein-Rich Legumes
Dinner	Smoothie: Cultured Coconut Milk, Raspberries, Avocado and Collard Greens

Side: Chickpeas With Cumin and Lemon (Boiled Tender, then Tossed with Ground Cumin, Ginger, and Fresh Lemon Juice). | Immune Boost |

Table 2.21: March - Sunday

Meal	Menu	Notes
Breakfast	Juice: Carrots, Celery, Cucumber, Spinach, Lemon + Chickpea Protein	Detox Support
Lunch	Salad: Kale + Omena, Romaine Lettuce, Cucumber, Green Onions and Cherry Tomato	Iron-Rich Protein
Dinner	Smoothie: Almond Milk, Blueberries and Baby Kale

Side: Red Lentils with Ginger and Celery (Simmered until Creamy with Grated Ginger, Coriander, and Leek Greens). | Anti-Inflammatory Dinner |

March Recap

March emphasized balance of treadmill exercise and healing nutrition. Legumes (lentils, chickpeas, cannellini, black-eyed peas), salmon, omena, and chicken ensured protein targets were met. Leafy greens, berries, chia/hemp, and turmeric strengthened anti-inflammatory protection.

Monthly Meal Plans After My Breast Cancer Treatment: April

This April plan continued the rhythm of daily healing meals, rich in leafy greens, legumes, fish, and chicken. I stayed consistent with portion sizes and anti-inflammatory foods. This month's plan reflects the discipline that stabilized my energy and maintained gut health.

Table 2.22: April - Monday

Meal	Menu	Notes
Breakfast	Juice: Carrots, Celery, Cucumber, Kale, Lemon + Pea Protein	Add Psyllium Husk
Lunch	Spinach & Arugula Salad + Boiled Mung Beans, Cucumber, Cherry Tomato and Herbs	Orange Juice Dressing
Dinner	Smoothie: Almond Yogurt, Spinach, Strawberries and Chia Side: Black-Eyed Peas with Ginger and Cumin (Boiled Soft and Tossed with Ginger, Cumin, and a Sprinkle of Parsley).	Light, Anti-Inflammatory

Table 2.23: April - Tuesday

Meal	Menu	Notes
Breakfast	Juice: Celery, Cucumber, Spinach, Kiwi, Ginger + Chickpea Protein	Kiwi for Vitamin C
Lunch	Salad: Kale + Salmon, Cucumber, Tomato and Arugula	Steam or Bake Covered, No Charring
Dinner	Smoothie: Almond Milk, Chopped and Steamed White Cabbage and Strawberries Side: Green Peas with Mint and Basil (Lightly Steamed and finished with Chopped Mint and Basil).	Supports Hormone Balance

Table 2.24: April - Wednesday

Meal	Menu	Notes
Breakfast	Juice: Carrots, Cucumber, Kale, Beetroot, Lemon, Ginger + Mung Bean Protein	Beet Supports Blood Levels
Lunch	Salad: Spinach + Chickpeas, Cucumber, Red Onion, Tomato and Herbs	Citrus Dressing
Dinner	Smoothie: Almond Milk, Raspberries, Lettuce and Chia Side: Pigeon Peas with Basil and Lime (Boiled until tender, then Brightened with Basil and a Squeeze of Lime.	Antioxidant-Rich

Table 2.25: April - Thursday

Meal	Menu	Notes
Breakfast	Juice: Celery, Cucumber, Kale, Green Apple Skin, Ginger + Chickpea Protein	Fiber from Apple Skin
Lunch	Salad: Spinach + Hard Organic Chicken, Cucumber, Tomato, Carrots	Protein Dense; No Oil Frying
Dinner	Smoothie: Almond Milk, Blueberries, Banana, Hemp Seeds and Collard Greens

Side: Lentils with Turmeric and Parsley (Cooked with, Celery, and Turmeric; Topped with Chopped Parsley). | Anti-Inflammatory Blend |

Table 2.26: April - Friday

Meal	Menu	Notes
Breakfast	Juice: Carrots, Celery, Cucumber, Spinach Leaves, Lemon + Mung Bean Protein	Balanced Breakfast I always add Cinnamon, Turmeric and Black Pepper
Lunch	Salad: Arugula + Cannellini Beans, Cucumber, Tomato, Bell Pepper	White Beans for Protein & Fiber
Dinner	Smoothie: Almond Milk, Blackberries, Green Apple Peels and Collard Greens.

Side: Baked Hard Chicken; Kienyeji (Boiled until Tender with Celery and Leek Greens, then Baked or Air-Fried with Thyme, Coriander, and a Squeeze of Lemon). | Gut-Healing Focus |

Table 2.27: April - Saturday

Meal	Menu	Notes
Breakfast	Juice: Carrots, Cucumber, Kale, Kiwi, Ginger + Pea Protein	Vitamin C-Rich Juice
Lunch	Salad: Spinach + Black-Eyed Peas, Cucumber, Tomato and Herbs	Protein-Rich Legumes
Dinner	Smoothie: Almond Milk, Raspberries, Hemp Seeds, Mixed Leafy Greens and Orange Side: Mung Beans with Ginger and Herbs (Cooked or Lightly Sprouted, then Mixed with Ginger and Chopped Coriander).	Immune Boost

Table 2.28: April - Sunday

Meal	Menu	Notes
Breakfast	Juice: Carrots, Celery, Cucumber, Spinach, Lemon + Chickpea Protein	Detox Support
Lunch	Salad: Chopped Kale + Omena, Beet Greens, Cucumber, Tomato and Red Onions	Iron-Rich Protein
Dinner	Smoothie: Almond Milk, Blueberries, Chia and Banana and Arugula Side: Mixed Beans with Herbs and Lime (Kidney, Black, and White Beans Boiled Soft, Tossed with Celery, Cilantro, and Lime Juice).	Anti-Inflammatory Dinner

April Recap

April's nutrition focused on consistency and balance: leafy greens, beans (mung, chickpeas, cannellini, black-eyed peas), fish (salmon, omena), and hard organic chicken. Anti-inflammatory boosters included turmeric, ginger, chia/hemp, and berries. This diet stabilized gut health while supporting recovery and strength

Monthly Meal Plans After My Breast Cancer Treatment: May

This May plan kept meals structured, nutrient-dense, and consistent. It balanced lean proteins, leafy greens, legumes, and anti-inflammatory foods, ensuring sustained recovery and strength.

Table 2.35: May - Monday

Meal	Menu	Notes
Breakfast	Juice: Carrots, Celery, Cucumber, Kale, Ginger, Lemon + Pea Protein	Add Psyllium Husk if Desired
Lunch	Salad: Spinach + Mung Beans, Red Onion, Cherry Tomato, Avocado and Herbs	Dressed with Citrus Juice
Dinner	Smoothie: Almond Milk, Spinach, Blueberries, Chia Seeds, Green Apple Peels and Watermelon Side: White Beans with Parsley and Turmeric (Soft-Cooked, then Tossed with Turmeric, Celery and Parsley).	Antioxidant Blend

Table 2.30: May - Tuesday

Meal	Menu	Notes
Breakfast	Juice: Celery, Cucumber, Red Cabbage, Kiwi, Ginger, Lemon + Chickpea Protein	Kiwi adds Vitamin C
Lunch	Salad: Kale + Salmon, Cucumber, Cherry Tomato, Yellow Bell Pepper and Red Onion	Bake Salmon, No Charring
Dinner	Smoothie: Almond Milk, Strawberries, Hemp Seeds and Spinach Side: Mung Beans with Ginger and Herbs (Cooked or Lightly Sprouted, then Mixed with Ginger and Chopped Coriander).	Hormone Support

Table 2.31: May - Wednesday

Meal	Menu	Notes
Breakfast	Juice: Carrots, Cucumber, Kale Leaves, Beetroot, Lemon, 1-Inch Ginger + Mung Protein	Beet Supports Blood Health
Lunch	Salad: Arugula + Chickpeas, Grated Carrots, Cherry Tomato, Herbs and Avocado	Citrus Dressing
Dinner	Smoothie: Almond Milk, Raspberries, Chia Seeds and Spinach and Banana Side: Black-Eyed Peas with Ginger and Cumin (Boiled Soft and Tossed with Ginger, Cumin, and a Sprinkle of Parsley).	Antioxidant Boost

Table 2.32: May - Thursday

Meal	Menu	Notes
Breakfast	Juice: Celery Stalks, Cucumber, Red Cabbage, Green Apple Skin, Lemon, Ginger + Chickpea Protein	Fiber From Apple Skin
Lunch	Salad: Kale + Hard Organic Chicken, Cherry Tomato and Green Onion	Protein-Dense, No Oil Frying
Dinner	Smoothie: Almond Milk, Blueberries, Hemp Seeds and Lettuce Side: Red Lentils with Ginger and Celery (Simmered until Creamy with Grated Ginger, Coriander, and Leek Greens).	Anti-Inflammatory Dinner

Table 2.33: May - Friday

Meal	Menu	Notes
Breakfast	Juice: Carrots, Celery, Cucumber, Kale, Ginger, Lemon + Mung Protein	Balanced Breakfast
Lunch	Salad: Arugula + Cannellini Beans, Cucumber, Tomato, Green Onion and Bell Pepper	Fiber-Rich Legumes
Dinner	Smoothie: Almond Milk, Blackberries, Chia Seeds, Spinach and Banana Side: Lentils with Turmeric and Parsley (Cooked with Cumin, Celery, Black Pepper and Turmeric; Topped with Chopped Parsley).	Gut Support

Table 2.34: May - Saturday

Meal	Menu	Notes
Breakfast	Juice: Carrots, Beetroot, Cucumber, Kale, Kiwi, Lemon, Ginger + Pea Protein	Vitamin C Boost
Lunch	Salad: Spinach + Black-Eyed Peas, Green Onion, Cucumber, Cherry Tomato, Avocado and Herbs	Protein F from Legumes
Dinner	Smoothie: Almond Milk, Raspberries, Hemp Seeds, Green Apple Skin and Collard Greens Side: Green Peas with Mint and Basil (Lightly Steamed and Finished with Chopped Mint and Basil).	Immune Boost

Table 2.35: May - Sunday

Meal	Menu	Notes
Breakfast	Juice: Carrots, Celery, Cucumber, While Cabbage, Ginger, Lemon + Chickpea Protein	Detox Support
Lunch	Salad: Kale + Omena, Red Onion, Avocado and Tomato	Iron-Rich Protein
Dinner	Smoothie: Almond Milk, Arugula, Blueberries and Banana Side: Pigeon Peas with Basil and Lime (Boiled until tender, then Brightened with Basil and a Squeeze of Lime).	Anti-Inflammatory Blend

May Recap

May continued with rotation of legumes (mung, chickpeas, cannellini, black-eyed peas), proteins (salmon, omena, chicken), and leafy greens (kale, spinach, arugula). Anti-inflammatory focus remained strong with turmeric, chia/hemp, and berries.

Monthly Meal Plans After My Breast Cancer Treatment: June

This June plan emphasized consistency with nutrient-rich juices, salads, and smoothies. It maintained high-protein legumes, lean fish and chicken, and anti-inflammatory foods for strength and vitality.

Table 2.36: June - Monday

Meal	Menu	Notes
Breakfast	Juice: Carrots, Celery, Cucumber, Kale, Ginger, Lemon + Pea Protein	Add Psyllium Husk if Desired
Lunch	Salad: Spinach + Lentils, Cucumber, Tomato, Avocado and Herbs	Dressed with Citrus Juice
Dinner	Smoothie: Almond Milk, Collard Greens, Blueberries, Chia Seeds and Banana Side: White Beans with Parsley and Turmeric (Soft-Cooked, then Tossed with Turmeric, Celery and Parsley).	Antioxidant Blend

Table 2.37: June - Tuesday

Meal	Menu	Notes
Breakfast	Juice: Celery, Carrots, Cucumber, Red Cabbage, Kiwi, Lemon, Ginger + Chickpea Protein	Kiwi Adds Vitamin C
Lunch	Salad: Kale + Salmon, Cucumber, Tomato and Green Onion	Bake Salmon, No Charring
Dinner	Smoothie: Almond Milk, Strawberries, Steamed Spinach and Hemp Seeds

Side: Cannellini Beans with Celery and Lemon (Boiled until Creamy, finished with Celery, Thyme, and Lemon Zest. | Hormone Support |

Table 2.38: June - Wednesday

Meal	Menu	Notes
Breakfast	Juice: Carrots, Cucumber, Kale, Beetroot, Lemon, Ginger + Mung Protein	Beet Supports Blood Health
Lunch	Salad: Red Cabbage + Chickpeas, Cucumber, Tomato, Avocado and Herbs	Citrus Dressing
Dinner	Smoothie: Almond Milk, Spinach, Raspberries, Banana and Chia Seeds
Side:	Antioxidant Boost I add banana to make the smoothie taste better for me. The healthy sugar does not rush to the bloodstream.

Table 2.39: June - Thursday

Meal	Menu	Notes
Breakfast	Juice: Celery, Cucumber, Kale, Green Apple Skin, Lemon, Ginger + Chickpea Protein	Fiber From Apple Skin
Lunch	Salad: Arugula + Hard Organic Chicken, Cherry Tomato and Red Onions	Protein-Dense, No Oil Frying
Dinner	Smoothie: Almond Yogurt, Blueberries, Hemp Seeds, Watermelon and Spinach Side: Mung Beans with Ginger and Herbs (Cooked or Lightly Sprouted, then Mixed with Ginger and Chopped Coriander).	Anti-Inflammatory Dinner

Table 2.40: June - Friday

Meal	Menu	Notes
Breakfast	Juice: Carrots, Celery, Cucumber, White Cabbage, Ginger, Lemon + Mung Protein	Balanced Breakfast I never forget to add Cinnamon
Lunch	Salad: Arugula + Cannellini Beans, Green Onion, Tomato and Bell Pepper	Fiber-Rich Legumes
Dinner	Smoothie: Almond Milk, Blackberries, Spinach, Fresh Squeezed Orange Juice and Avocado Side: Chickpeas with Cumin and Lemon (Boiled until tender, then Seasoned with Ground Cumin, Ginger, and Fresh Lemon Juice).	Gut Support

Table 2.41: June - Saturday

Meal	Menu	Notes
Breakfast	Juice: Carrots, Cucumber, Beetroot, Kale, Kiwi, Ginger + Pea Protein	Vitamin C Boost
Lunch	Salad: Mixed Greens + Black-Eyed Peas, Cherry Tomato, Green Onion and Herbs	Protein from Legumes My Legumes are always Boiled for Salad
Dinner	Smoothie: Almond Milk, Raspberries, Hemp Seeds, Spinach and Avocado Side: Red Lentils with Ginger and Celery (Simmered until Creamy with Grated Ginger, Coriander and Leek Greens).	Immune Boost

Table 2.42: June - Sunday

Meal	Menu	Notes
Breakfast	Juice: Carrots, Celery, Cucumber, Collard Greens, Ginger, Lemon + Chickpea Protein	Detox Support
Lunch	Salad: Kale + Omena, Red Onion, Tomato and Avocado	Iron-Rich Protein
Dinner	Smoothie: Almond Milk, Blueberries, Chia Seeds, Watermelon and Spinach Side: Lentils with Turmeric and Parsley (Cooked with Cummin, Celery, Black Pepper and Turmeric; Topped with Chopped Parsley).	Anti-Inflammatory Blend

June Recap

June continued steady healing nutrition with legumes (lentils, chickpeas, cannellini, black-eyed peas), fish (salmon, omena), and chicken. Leafy greens, turmeric, chia/hemp, and berries kept the anti-inflammatory focus strong.

Monthly Meal Plans After My Breast Cancer Treatment: July

This July plan focused on maintaining a lean, nutrient-rich routine with juices, salads, and smoothies. Meals emphasized high protein, fiber, and anti-inflammatory foods to sustain energy and strength.

Table 2.43: July - Monday

Meal	Menu	Notes
Breakfast	Juice: Carrots, Celery, Cucumber, Kale, Ginger, Lemon + Pea Protein	Add Psyllium Husk If Desired
Lunch	Salad: Arugula + Mung Beans, Bell Peppers, Cherry Tomato, Herbs and Avocado	Dressed with Citrus Juice
Dinner	Smoothie: Almond Milk, Spinach, Blueberries, Banana and Chia Seeds Side: Red Lentils with Ginger and Celery (Simmered until Creamy with Grated Ginger, Coriander, and Leek Greens).	Anti-Inflammatory Blend

Table 2.44: July - Tuesday

Meal	Menu	Notes
Breakfast	Juice: Celery, Carrots, Cucumber, Red Cabbage, Kiwi, Lemon, Ginger + Chickpea Protein	Kiwi Adds Vitamin C
Lunch	Salad: Kale + Salmon, Red Onion, Cherry Tomato, Red Bell Peppers	Bake Salmon, No Charring
Dinner	Smoothie: Almond Milk, Spinach, Strawberries and Hemp Seeds Side: Black-Eyed Peas with Ginger and Cumin (Boiled Soft and Tossed with Ginger, Cumin, and a Sprinkle of Parsley).	Hormone Support

Table 2.45: July - Wednesday

Meal	Menu	Notes
Breakfast	Juice: Carrots, Cucumber, Kale, Beetroot, Lemon, Ginger + Mung Protein	Beet Supports Blood Health
Lunch	Salad: Spinach + Chickpeas, Bell Peppers, Cherry Tomatoes, Avocado and Herbs	Citrus Dressing
Dinner	Smoothie: Almond Milk, Collard Greens, Raspberries, Watermelon and Chia Seeds Side: Mung Beans with Ginger and Herbs (Cooked or Lightly Sprouted, then Mixed with Ginger and Chopped Coriander).	Antioxidant Boost

Table 2.46: July - Thursday

Meal	Menu	Notes
Breakfast	Juice: Carrots, Celery, Cucumber, Kale, Green Apple Skin, Lemon, Ginger + Chickpea Protein	Fiber From Apple Skin
Lunch	Salad: Spinach + Hard Organic Chicken, Green Onion and Cherry Tomatoes Fruit: Tangerine	Protein-Dense, No Oil Frying
Dinner	Smoothie: Almond Milk, Blueberries, Hemp Seed, Watermelon and Arugula Side: Pigeon Peas with Basil and Lime (Boiled until tender, then Brightened with Basil and a Squeeze of Lime).	Anti-Inflammatory Dinner

Table 2.47: July - Friday

Meal	Menu	Notes
Breakfast	Juice: Carrots, Beetroot, Cucumber, Red Cabbage, Ginger, Lemon + Mung Beans Protein	Balanced Breakfast
Lunch	Salad: Arugula + Cannellini Beans, Green Onions, Cherry Tomatoes, Bell Pepper and Avocado	Fiber-Rich Legumes
Dinner	Smoothie: Almond Milk, Blackberries, Chia Seeds, Spinach and Banana Side: Chickpeas with Cumin and Lemon (Boiled until tender, then Seasoned with Ground Cumin, Ginger and Fresh Lemon Juice).	Gut Support

Table 2.48: July - Saturday

Meal	Menu	Notes
Breakfast	Juice: Carrots, Celery, Cucumber, Kale, Kiwi, Lemon, Ginger + Pea Protein	Vitamin C Boost
Lunch	Salad: Spinach Salad + Black-Eyed Peas, Bell Peppers, Tomato, Avocado and Herbs	Protein from Legumes
Dinner	Smoothie: Almond Milk, Raspberries, Hemp Seeds, Collard Greens and Freshly Squeezed Orange Juice Side: Green Peas with Mint and Basil (Lightly Steamed and finished with Chopped Mint and Basil).	Immune Boost

Table 2.49: July - Sunday

Meal	Menu	Notes
Breakfast	Juice: Carrots, Beetroot, Cucumber, Red Cabbage, Ginger, Lemon + Chickpea Protein	Detox Support
Lunch	Salad: Lettuce + Omena, Red Onion and Cherry Tomato	Iron-Rich Protein
Dinner	Smoothie: Almond Milk, Blueberries, Watermelon, Chia Seeds and Spinach Side: Pigeon Peas with Basil and Lime (Boiled until tender, then Brightened with Basil and a Squeeze of Lime).	Anti-Inflammatory Blend

July Recap

July sustained the rhythm of healing nutrition: legumes (mung, chickpeas, cannellini, black-eyed peas), fish (salmon, omena), and chicken formed the protein base. Leafy greens, turmeric, chia/hemp, and berries kept inflammation low and energy stable.

Monthly Meal Plans After My Breast Cancer Treatment: August

This August plan reflects continued structure in healing nutrition with detailed daily meals. It also introduces my experience with fresh wheatgrass juice, which I began two months after chemotherapy with guidance from my oncologist and oncology dieticians. I planted wheatgrass at home in trays with only water, juicing it fresh to obtain chlorophyll. This became an important addition to my morning routine.

Table 2.50: August - Monday

Meal	Menu	Notes
Breakfast	Juice: Carrots, Celery, Cucumber, Kale, Ginger, Lemon + Pea Protein	I prefer this breakfast as it is easy to prepare. I take it right after working out.
Lunch	Salad: Spinach + Mung Beans, Cucumber, Tomato, Herbs and Avocado	Orange Juice Dressing
Dinner	Smoothie: Almond Milk, Spinach, Blueberries and Fresh Juiced Orange Side: Baked Hard Chicken; Kienyeji (Boiled until tender with Celery and Leek Greens, then Baked or Air-Fried with Thyme, Coriander and a Squeeze of Lemon).	Anti-Inflammatory Blend

Table 2.51: August - Tuesday

Meal	Menu	Notes
Breakfast	Juice: Carrots, Celery, Cucumber, Kale, Kiwi, Lemon, Ginger + Chickpea Protein	Kiwi Adds Vitamin C
Lunch	Salad: Arugula + Salmon, Green Onion and Cherry Tomato. Fruit: Orange	Steam or Bake Salmon, No Charring
Dinner	Smoothie: Almond Milk, Strawberries, Hemp Seeds, Spinach and Watermelon Side: Green Peas with Mint and Basil (Lightly Steamed and finished with Chopped Mint and Basil).	Hormone Support

Table 2.52: August - Wednesday

Meal	Menu	Notes
Breakfast	Juice: Carrots, Cucumber, Kale, Beetroot, Lemon, Ginger + Mung Protein	Beet Supports Blood Health
Lunch	Salad: Arugula + Chickpeas, Cherry Tomatoes, Herbs	Citrus Dressing
Dinner	Smoothie: Almond Milk, Steamed Spinach, Raspberries, Chia Seeds and Bell Peppers Side: Pigeon Peas with Basil and Lime (Boiled until tender, then Brightened with Basil and a Squeeze of Lime).	Antioxidant Boost

Table 2.53: August - Thursday

Meal	Menu	Notes
Breakfast	Juice: Celery, Cucumber, Kale, Green Apple Skin, Ginger, Lemon + Chickpea Protein	Fiber From Apple Skin
Lunch	Salad: Spinach + Hard Organic Chicken, Red Bell Peppers, Cherry Tomatoes and Green Onions	Protein-Dense, No Oil Frying
Dinner	Smoothie: Almond Milk, Blueberries, Lettuce, Green Apple Peels and Hemp Seeds Side: Red Lentils with Ginger and Celery (Simmered until Creamy with Grated Ginger, Coriander, and Leek Greens).	Anti-Inflammatory Dinner

Table 2.54: August - Friday

Meal	Menu	Notes
Breakfast	Juice: Carrots, Celery, Cucumber, Spinach, Lemon + Mung Protein	Balanced Breakfast
Lunch	Salad: Arugula + Cannellini Beans, Red Onions, Cherry Tomatoes and Bell Pepper	Fiber-Rich Legumes
Dinner	Smoothie: Almond Milk, Blackberries, Chia Side: Baked Hard Chicken; Kienyeji (Boiled until tender with Celery and Leek Greens, Then Baked or Air-Fried with Thyme, Coriander, and a Squeeze of Lemon).	Gut Support

Table 2.55: August - Saturday

Meal	Menu	Notes
Breakfast	Juice: Carrots, Cucumber, Kale, Kiwi, Ginger + Pea Protein	Vitamin C Boost
Lunch	Salad: Spinach Salad + Black-Eyed Peas, Cucumber, Green Onions, Cherry Tomato and Herbs	Protein from Legumes
Dinner	Smoothie: Almond Milk, Raspberries, Green Apple Peels, Hemp Seed and Lettuce Side: Baked Wild Salmon with Herbs (Seasoned with Rosemary, Thyme, Grated Ginger and Lemon Zest, then Baked or Air-Fried in Parchment for a Clean, Refreshing Flavor).	Immune Boost

Table 2.56: August - Sunday

Meal	Menu	Notes
Breakfast	Juice: Carrots, Celery, Cucumber, Spinach, Lemon + Chickpea Protein	Detox Support
Lunch	Salad: Red Cabbage + Omena, Cucumber, Green Onions and Tomato	Iron-Rich Protein
Dinner	Smoothie: Almond Milk, Blueberries, Kale and Chia Side: Pigeon Peas with Basil and Lime (Boiled until tender, then Brightened with Basil and a Squeeze of Lime).	Anti-Inflammatory Blend

August Recap

August strengthened healing with the inclusion of fresh wheatgrass juice, providing chlorophyll and added anti-inflammatory benefits. Legumes (mung, chickpeas, cannellini, black-eyed peas), fish (salmon, omena), and chicken remained protein staples. Leafy greens, turmeric, chia/hemp, and berries kept the anti-inflammatory focus strong.

Monthly Meal Plans After My Breast Cancer Treatment: September

This September plan sustained my rhythm of healing nutrition, keeping meals simple, plant-forward, and protein-rich. It emphasized variety with legumes, leafy greens, fish, and chicken, ensuring balance while keeping inflammation low.

Table 2.57: September - Monday

Meal	Menu	Notes
Breakfast	Juice: Carrots, Celery, Cucumber, Kale, Lemon, Ginger + Pea Protein	Add Psyllium Husk If Desired
Lunch	Salad: Arugula + Lentils, Green Onion, Cherry Tomato and Herbs	Citrus Dressing
Dinner	Smoothie: Almond Milk, Spinach, Kiwi, Orange, Chia Seeds Side: Baked Hard Chicken; Kienyeji (Boiled until tender with Celery and Leek Greens, then Baked or Air-Fried with Thyme, Coriander, a Squeeze of Lemon)	Antioxidant Blend The spinach I use for smoothies is mostly steamed

Table 2.58: September - Tuesday

Meal	Menu	Notes
Breakfast	Juice: Carrots, Celery, Cucumber, Spinach, Orange, Ginger + Lemon and Chickpea Protein	Kiwi Adds Vitamin C
Lunch	Salad: Kale + Salmon, Red Onion and Tomato	Bake Salmon, No Charring
Dinner	Smoothie: Almond Milk, Strawberries, Hemp Seed and Lettuce Side: Mixed Beans with Herbs and Lime (Kidney, Black and White Beans Boiled Soft, Tossed with Celery, Cilantro and Lime Juice).	Hormone Support

Table 2.59: September - Wednesday

Meal	Menu	Notes
Breakfast	Juice: Carrots, Cucumber, Kale, Beetroot, Lemon, Ginger + Mung Protein	Beetroot Supports Blood Health
Lunch	Salad: Spinach + Chickpeas, Tomato, Green Onions, Avocado and Herbs	Citrus Dressing
Dinner	Smoothie: Almond Milk, Raspberries, Green Apple Peels, Arugula and Chia Side: Cannellini Beans with Celery and Lemon (Boiled until Creamy, finished with Celery, Thyme, and Lemon Zest).	Antioxidant Boost

Table 2.60: September - Thursday

Meal	Menu	Notes
Breakfast	Juice: Celery, Cucumber, Carrots, Kale, Green Apple Skin, Lemon, Ginger + Chickpea Protein	Fiber From Apple Skin
Lunch	Salad: Spinach + Hard Organic Chicken, Tomato,	Protein-Dense, No Oil Frying
Dinner	Smoothie: Almond Milk, Collard Greens, Blueberries, Banana and Avocado Side: Pigeon Peas with Basil and Lime (Boiled until tender, then brightened with Basil and a Squeeze of Lime).	Anti-Inflammatory Dinner

Table 2.61: September - Friday

Meal	Menu	Notes
Breakfast	Juice: Carrots, Celery, Cucumber, Red Cabbage, Lemon, Ginger + Mung Protein	Balanced Breakfast
Lunch	Salad: Arugula + Cannellini Beans, Cucumber, Cherry Tomato, Green Onion, Bell Pepper and Avocado	Fiber-Rich Legumes
Dinner	Smoothie: Almond Milk Yogurt, Blueberries, Chia Seeds and Fresh Orange Juice Side: Red Lentils with Ginger and Celery (Simmered until Creamy with Grated Ginger, Coriander and Leek Greens).	Gut Support

Table 2.62: September - Saturday

Meal	Menu	Notes
Breakfast	Juice: Carrots, Cucumber, Kale, Kiwi, Ginger, Beetroot, Lemon + Pea Protein	Vitamin C Boost
Lunch	Salad: Spinach + Black-Eyed Peas, Red and Yellow Bell Peppers, Cherry Tomato, Green Onions and Herbs	Protein from Legumes
Dinner	Smoothie: Almond Milk, Raspberries, Lettuce, Orange, Hemp Seeds Side: Mung Beans with Ginger and Herbs (Cooked or Lightly Sprouted, then Mixed with Ginger and Chopped Coriander).	Immune Boost

Table 2.63: September - Sunday

Meal	Menu	Notes
Breakfast	Juice: Carrots, Celery, Cucumber, Red Cabbage, Ginger, Lemon + Chickpea Protein	Detox Support
Lunch	Salad: Kale + Omena, Bell Peppers, Green Onion and Tomato	Iron-Rich Protein Refer to Salad Omena Recipe
Dinner	Smoothie: Almond Milk, Blueberries, Chia Seeds and Spinach Side: Red Lentils with Ginger and Celery (Simmered until Creamy with Grated Ginger, Coriander, and Leek Greens).	Anti-Inflammatory Blend

September Recap

September sustained healing nutrition with consistent rotation of legumes (lentils, chickpeas, cannellini, black-eyed peas), fish (salmon, omena), and chicken. Leafy greens, turmeric, chia/hemp, and berries maintained an anti-inflammatory foundation

Monthly Meal Plans After My Breast Cancer Treatment: October

This October plan reflects my ongoing healing nutrition with consistent structure: juices, leafy salads, and smoothies rich in protein, fiber, and anti-inflammatory foods. This month sustained the core practices that supported recovery and energy.

Table 2.64: October - Monday

Meal	Menu	Notes
Breakfast	Juice: Carrots, Celery, Kale, Lemon, Ginger + Pea Protein	Add Psyllium Husk if Desired. Great for Fiber
Lunch	Salad: Arugula + Mung Beans, Cucumber, Red Onion, Cherry Tomato and Herbs	Dressed with Citrus Juice
Dinner	Smoothie: Almond Milk, Spinach, Blueberries, Orange and Avocado Side: Pigeon Peas with Basil and Lime (Boiled until tender, then brightened with Basil and a Squeeze of Lime).	Anti-Inflammatory Blend

Table 2.65: October - Tuesday

Meal	Menu	Notes
Breakfast	Juice: Celery, Cucumber, Kale, Kiwi, Ginger, Lemon + Chickpea Protein	Kiwi Adds Vitamin C
Lunch	Salad: Spinach + Salmon, Red Onion and Cherry Tomato Fruit: Strawberries	Bake Salmon, No Charring I literally eat spinach each day because of how rich in protein it is
Dinner	Smoothie: Cultured Coconut Milk, Goji Berries, Hemp Seeds and Collard Greens Side: Mixed Beans with Herbs and Lime (Pinto and White Beans Boiled Soft, Tossed with Celery, Cilantro, and Lime Juice).	

Table 2.66: October - Wednesday

Meal	Menu	Notes
Breakfast	Juice: Carrots, Cucumber, White Cabbage, Beetroot, Lemon, Ginger + Mung Protein	Beet Supports Blood Health
Lunch	Salad: Spinach + Chickpeas, Bell Peppers, Cherry Tomato and Herbs	Citrus Dressing
Dinner	Smoothie: Almond Milk, Raspberries, Banana, Chia Seeds and Green Apple Peels Side: Green Peas with Mint and Basil (Lightly Steamed and finished With Chopped Mint and Basil).	Antioxidant Boost

Table 2.67: October - Thursday

Meal	Menu	Notes
Breakfast	Juice: Carrots, Celery, Cucumber, Kale, Green Apple Skin, Ginger + Chickpea Protein	Fiber From Apple Skin
Lunch	Salad: Mixed Greens + Hard Organic Chicken, Green Onions, Red Bell Peppers and Cherry Tomato	Protein-Dense, No Oil Frying
Dinner	Smoothie: Almond Milk, Blueberries, Hemp Seeds, Fresh Juiced Orange, Banana and Arugula Side: Cannellini Beans with Celery and Lemon (Boiled until creamy, finished with Celery, Thyme, and Lemon Zest).	Anti-Inflammatory Dinner

Table 2.68: October - Friday

Meal	Menu	Notes
Breakfast	Juice: Carrots, Beetroot, Cucumber, Red Cabbage, Lemon, Ginger + Mung Protein	Balanced Breakfast
Lunch	Salad: Arugula + Cannellini Beans, Tomato, Red Bell Pepper	Fiber-Rich Legumes
Dinner	Smoothie: Almond Milk, Blackberries, Green Apple Peels, Chia Seeds and Kale Side: Black-Eyed Peas with Ginger and Cumin (Boiled Soft and Tossed with Ginger, Cumin, and a Sprinkle of Parsley).	Gut Support

Table 2.69: October - Saturday

Meal	Menu	Notes
Breakfast	Juice: Carrots, Cucumber, Kale, Kiwi, Ginger, Beetroot, Lemon + Pea Protein	Vitamin C Boost
Lunch	Spinach Salad + Black-Eyed Peas, Red Onion, Cherry Tomato and Herbs	Protein From Legumes
Dinner	Smoothie: Almond Yogurt, Raspberries, Collard Greens and Strawberries Side: Steamed Hard Chicken with Parsley and Celery (Steamed to Retain Flavor, then Topped with Fresh Parsley, Celery and Lime Juice).	Immune Boost

Table 2.70: October - Sunday

Meal	Menu	Notes
Breakfast	Juice: Carrots, Celery, Cucumber, Red Cabbage, Ginger, Lemon + Chickpea Protein	Detox Support
Lunch	Salad: Kale + Omena, Cucumber, Cherry Tomato, Red Onion and Avocado	Iron-Rich Protein
Dinner	Smoothie: Almond Milk, Blueberries, Banana, Chia Seeds and Spinach Side: Mung Beans with Ginger and Herbs (Cooked or Lightly Sprouted, then Mixed with Ginger and Chopped Coriander).	Anti-Inflammatory Blend

October Recap

October sustained my healing nutrition with legumes (mung, chickpeas, cannellini, black-eyed peas), fish (salmon, omena), and chicken. Leafy greens daily, chia/hemp, turmeric, and berries helped maintain energy and reduce inflammation.

Monthly Meal Plans After My Breast Cancer Treatment: November

This November plan remained focused on clean, plant-rich meals with steady protein rotation. It helped sustain strength, supported bone and joint health, and kept inflammation low.

Table 2.71: November - Monday

Meal	Menu	Notes
Breakfast	Juice: Carrots, Celery, Cucumber, Kale, Lemon + Pea Protein	Add Psyllium Husk if Desired
Lunch	Salad: Red Cabbage + Boiled Mung Beans, Cucumber, Tomato, Green Onions and Herbs	Dressed with Citrus Juice
Dinner	Smoothie: Almond Milk, Spinach, Blueberries and Strawberries Side: Baked wild Salmon with Herbs (Seasoned with Rosemary, Thyme, Grated Ginger, and Lemon Zest, then Baked or Air-Fried in Parchment for a Clean, Refreshing Flavor.	Anti-Inflammatory Blend

Table 2.72: November - Tuesday

Meal	Menu	Notes
Breakfast	Juice: Celery, Cucumber, Spinach, Kiwi, Ginger + Chickpea Protein	Kiwi adds Vitamin C
Lunch	Salad: Kale + Salmon, Tomato and Red Onion	Bake Salmon, No Charring
Dinner	Smoothie: Almond Milk, Strawberries, Hemp Seeds and Arugula Side: Mixed Beans with Herbs and Lime (Kidney, Black, and White Beans Boiled Soft, Tossed with Celery, Cilantro, and Lime Juice).	Hormone Support

Table 2.73: November - Wednesday

Meal	Menu	Notes
Breakfast	Juice: Carrots, Cucumber, Red Cabbage, Beetroot, Lemon, Ginger + Mung Protein	Beet Supports Blood Health
Lunch	Salad: Spinach + Chickpeas, Green Onion, Cherry Tomato, Herbs and Avocado	Citrus Dressing
Dinner	Smoothie: Almond Milk, Raspberries, Chia Seeds and Kale Side: Black-Eyed Peas with Ginger and Cumin (Boiled Soft and Tossed with Ginger, Cumin, and a Sprinkle of Parsley).	Antioxidant Boost

Table 2.74: November - Thursday

Meal	Menu	Notes
Breakfast	Juice: Celery, Carrots, Cucumber, Kale, Green Apple Skin, Ginger + Chickpea Protein	Fiber From Apple Skin
Lunch	Salad: Spinach + Hard Organic Chicken, Cucumber, Tomato, Green Onions and Shredded Carrots	Protein-Dense, No Oil Frying
Dinner	Smoothie: Almond Milk, Blueberries, Banana, Hemp Seeds and Lettuce Side: Mung Beans with Ginger and Herbs (Cooked or Lightly Sprouted, then Mixed with Ginger and Chopped Coriander).	Anti-Inflammatory Dinner

Table 2.75: November - Friday

Meal	Menu	Notes
Breakfast	Juice: Carrots, Beetroot, Cucumber, Ginger, Red Cabbage, Lemon + Mung Beans Protein	Balanced Breakfast
Lunch	Salad: Arugula + Cannellini Beans, Green Onion, Tomato, Bell Pepper and Avocado	Fiber-Rich Legumes
Dinner	Smoothie: Almond Milk, Blackberries, Green Apple Peels and Spinach Side: Pigeon Peas with Basil and Lime (Boiled until tender, then brightened with Basil and a Squeeze of Lime).	Gut Support

Table 2.76: November - Saturday

Meal	Menu	Notes
Breakfast	Juice: Carrots, Cucumber, Kale, Kiwi, Ginger, Beetroot + Pea Protein	Vitamin C Boost
Lunch	Salad: Spinach + Black-Eyed Peas, Cherry Tomato, Avocado and Herbs	Protein from Legumes
Dinner	Smoothie: Almond Milk, Kiwi, Hemp Seed and Arugula Side: Chickpeas with Cumin and Lemon (Boiled until tender, then Seasoned with Ground Cumin, Ginger, and Fresh Lemon Juice).	Immune Boost

Table 2.77: November - Sunday

Meal	Menu	Notes
Breakfast	Juice: Carrots, Celery, Cucumber, Spinach, Lemon + Chickpea Protein	Detox Support
Lunch	Salad: Kale + Omena, Red Onion, Cherry Tomato and Avocado	Iron-Rich Protein
Dinner	Smoothie: Almond Milk, Blueberries, Orange, Chia Seeds and Mixed Greens Side: Green Peas with Mint and Basil (Lightly Steamed and finished with Chopped Mint and Basil).	Anti-Inflammatory Blend

November Recap

November highlighted clean, steady nutrition with legumes (mung, chickpeas, cannellini, black-eyed peas), fish (salmon, omena), and chicken. Leafy greens, chia/hemp, turmeric, and berries supported bone health, energy, and resilience through anti-inflammatory nutrition.

Monthly Meal Plans After My Breast Cancer Treatment: December

This December plan closed the year with consistency, reflection, and strength. It carried forward the rhythm of juices, leafy salads, and smoothies, ensuring a full year of clean, healing nutrition that supported my recovery and thriving.

Table 7.78: December - Monday

Meal	Menu	Notes
Breakfast	Juice: Carrots, Celery, Cucumber, Kale, Lemon + Pea Protein	Add Psyllium Husk if Desired
Lunch	Salad: Spinach & Arugula + Mung Beans, Cucumber, Green Onions, Tomato and Herbs	Dressed with Citrus Juice Herbs: I alternate between Cilantro and Parsley a lot
Dinner	Smoothie: Almond Milk, Spinach, Banana, Blueberries and Chia Side: Red Lentils with Ginger and Celery (Simmered until Creamy with Grated Ginger, Coriander and Leek Greens).	Anti-Inflammatory Blend

Table 7.79: December - Tuesday

Meal	Menu	Notes
Breakfast	Juice: Celery, Cucumber, Spinach, Kiwi, Ginger + Chickpea Protein	Kiwi adds Vitamin C
Lunch	Salad: Kale + Salmon, Tomato and Red Onions	Steam/Bake Salmon, No Charring
Dinner	Smoothie: Almond Milk, Strawberries, Hemp Seeds and Collard Greens Side: Mixed Beans with Herbs and Lime (Pinto, Black and White Beans Boiled Soft, Tossed with Celery, Cilantro and Lime Juice).	Hormone Support

Table 7.80: December - Wednesday

Meal	Menu	Notes
Breakfast	Juice: Carrots, Cucumber, Kale, Beet, Lemon, Ginger + Mung Protein	Beet Supports Blood Health
Lunch	Salad: Lettuce + Chickpeas, Green Onions, Tomato and Herbs	Citrus Dressing
Dinner	Smoothie: Almond Milk, Raspberries, Spinach and Chia Side: Lentils with Turmeric and Parsley (Cooked with Celery, and Turmeric; topped with Chopped Parsley).	Antioxidant Boost

Table 7.81: December - Thursday

Meal	Menu	Notes
Breakfast	Juice: Celery Stalks, Carrots, Kale, Green Apple Skin, Ginger + Chickpea Protein	Fiber From Apple Skin
Lunch	Salad: Spinach + Hard Organic Chicken, Cucumber, Tomato, Carrots	Protein-Dense, No Oil Frying
Dinner	Smoothie: Almond Milk, Blueberries, Arugula and Hemp Seeds. Side: Green Peas with Mint and Basil (Lightly Steamed and Finished with Chopped Mint and Basil for a Clean, Soothing Side).	Anti-Inflammatory Dinner

Table 7.82: December - Friday

Meal	Menu	Notes
Breakfast	Juice: Carrots, Celery, Cucumber, Collard Greens, Ginger, Lemon + Mung Protein	Balanced Breakfast
Lunch	Salad: Arugula + Cannellini Beans, Cherry Tomato, Bell Pepper, Green Onion and Avocado	Fiber-Rich Legumes
Dinner	Smoothie: Almond Milk, Kiwi, Chia, Green Apple Peels and Kale Side: Lentils With Turmeric and Parsley (Cooked with Turmeric and Black Pepper; Topped with Chopped Parsley).	Gut Support

Table 7.83: December - Saturday

Meal	Menu	Notes
Breakfast	Juice: Carrots, Cucumber, Kale, Kiwi, Ginger + Pea Protein	Vitamin C Boost
Lunch	Spinach Salad + Black-Eyed Peas, Cucumber, Cherry Tomato, Red Onions and Herbs	Protein from Legumes
Dinner	Smoothie: Almond Milk, Raspberries, Green Apple Peels, Mixed Greens and Avocado Side: Chickpeas with Cumin and Lemon — Boiled until tender, then Seasoned with Ground Cumin, Ginger, and Fresh Lemon Juice.	Immune Boost

Table 7.84: December - Sunday

Meal	Menu	Notes
Breakfast	Juice: Carrots, Celery, Cucumber, Spinach, Lemon + Chickpea Protein	Detox Support
Lunch	Salad: White Cabbage + Omena, Red Onion and Tomato	Iron-Rich Protein
Dinner	Smoothie: Almond Yogurt, Blueberries, Arugula and Chia Seeds Side: Red Lentils with Ginger and Celery (Simmered until Creamy with Grated Ginger, Coriander, and Leek Greens).	Anti-Inflammatory Blend

December Recap

December closed the year with steady, structured nutrition: legumes (mung, chickpeas, cannellini, black-eyed peas), fish (salmon, omena), and chicken continued as protein staples. Leafy greens, chia/hemp, turmeric, and berries rounded out a year of consistent anti-inflammatory eating and thriving.

Kenyan Cultural Cancer Care Meal Plan

As a Kenyan, African, and immigrant in the United States, I understand that not everyone can easily follow the same meal plans I've shared earlier in this book. Food choices often reflect our culture, accessibility, and environment. Many of the foods and vegetables I use here in the United States may not be easily available in Kenya or other parts of Africa — just as some foods that are common and fresh in Kenya are difficult to find here.

Because of these differences, and from my experience working with cancer patients through my organization, I want to share a cultural weekly meal plan that I designed specifically for cancer patients in Kenya. This plan reflects our local foods and daily rhythms. It is meant to be practical, affordable, and culturally familiar, while still following the same nutritional principles that guided my own recovery.

This plan is tailored for patients undergoing active cancer treatment, which is why it prioritizes foods that are easy to digest, nutrient-dense, and gentle on the stomach while supporting blood count stability and tissue repair. The plan also accommodates limited access to refrigeration and specialty ingredients. It follows the same key principles outlined earlier in this book:

- Balanced proteins, healthy fats, and fiber-rich carbohydrates
- Natural anti-inflammatory foods
- Avoidance of refined oils, processed sugars, and heavily fried or charred meals
- Fresh, seasonal, locally grown produce wherever possible

Key Features of the Cultural Cancer Care Meal Plan

Protein Sources:

- Hard chicken (kienyeji), omena, eggs, lentils, beans, green grams (mung beans), pigeon peas, cowpeas.
- These are culturally familiar, high in iron and protein, and easy to incorporate into soups, stews, or porridge.

Carbohydrate Sources (Moderate Portions):

- Sweet potatoes, pumpkins, arrowroots, amaranth, millet porridge, or small portions of unpolished brown rice or sorghum ugali.
- Limit portions to match BMI-based requirements.

Vegetables:

- Emphasize leafy greens (kale, amaranth leaves, pumpkin leaves, managu, spinach), cruciferous vegetables (cabbage, cauliflower — only in small amounts for those with IBS), and anti-inflammatory additions like ginger, turmeric, garlic substitutes, and herbs.

Fruits:

- Focus on low-sugar, high-antioxidant fruits such as pawpaw (papaya), avocado, berries (if available), and citrus fruits.
- Avoid very sugary fruits like ripe bananas, mangoes, and grapes.

Healthy Fats:

- Use avocado, chia seeds, or sesame (in moderation).
- Avoid cooking oils when possible. For family meals, use a small amount of cold-pressed avocado oil.

Fluids:

- Hydrate consistently with clean warm water, herbal teas (ginger, lemongrass, moringa), and vegetable soups.
- Avoid fizzy, sugary, or colored drinks.

Final Note

This plan was created with a deep understanding of how nutrition, culture, and access intersect. Every meal respects the Kenyan palate and local food systems while maintaining the scientific foundation of cancer nutrition. It offers a bridge between medical dietary guidance and cultural identity a way to eat for healing without abandoning who we are.

While it was designed specifically for patients undergoing active treatment, it is also suitable for anyone who wants to live a healthier, cleaner lifestyle.

If you are not currently on treatment, you can still follow this plan by:

- Reducing your meals to three per day (breakfast, lunch, and dinner).
- Adjusting your portion sizes to match your daily activity level and BMI.
- Continuing to prioritize whole, plant-rich, and low-inflammatory foods as your everyday way of living.

This cultural plan reminds us that healing and health do not begin or end with illness — they are daily choices, made one mindful meal at a time.

Table 7.85: Kenya Cultural Cancer Patient Weekly Meal Plan

Day	Breakfast	Snack	Lunch	Snack	Dinner	Snack
Monday	Wimbi porridge, carrots, cashews, apple	Protein shake	Green bananas, spinach, kunde, beans, blue berries	Berries	Brown rice, lentils, peas, cabbage	Protein shake
Tuesday	Oatmeal porridge, steamed cabbage, berries	Protein shake	Millet ugali, omena, sukuma wiki, carrot, apple	Orange	Kienyeji vegetables (managu, mchicha), kidney beans	Protein shake
Wednesday	Slice of whole grain bread, carrots, 2 egg whites, papaya	Protein shake	Brown rice, cabbage, peas, lentils, avocado	Papaya	Sweet potatoes, lentils, spinach, cabbage	Protein shake
Thursday	Sweet potatoes, steamed cabbage, 2 egg whites, orange	Protein shake	Kidney beans, nduma, spinach, carrots, orange	Orange	Millet ugali, managu, mchicha, omena	Protein shake
Friday	Arrowroots, sukuma wiki, groundnuts, grapes	Protein shake	Sweet potatoes, lentils, spinach, cabbage, papaya	Avocado	Cabbage, carrots, chickpeas	Protein shake
Saturday	Oatmeal porridge, steamed cabbage, berries	Protein shake	Kienyeji vegetables (managu, pumpkin leaves), millet ugali, omena, apple	Berries	Brown rice, sukuma wiki, peas, lentils	Protein shake
Sunday	Slice of whole grain bread, carrots, 2 egg whites, papaya	Protein shake	Brown rice, organic chicken, peas, cabbage, orange	Orange	Spinach, beetroot, beans	Protein shake

PART THREE

Recipes & Practical Guides

After sharing my monthly meal plans, this section brings the practical side of my nutrition journey. These are the exact recipes I used, carefully measured, guided by oncology dieticians and nutritionists at one of the world's leading cancer treatment hospitals, and shaped by my personal needs during and after treatment.

The recipes are built on evidence-based nutrition principles: balancing protein, fiber, and natural anti-inflammatory foods. Each juice, smoothie, soup, or salad is portioned to match my BMI goals and healing process, with adjustments to protect gut health and reduce inflammation.

Here you will find:

- Juices that always include protein to prevent blood sugar spikes.
- Smoothies that served as my evening meals.
- Soft soups I relied on when I had mouth sores or needed anti-inflammatory comfort.
- Homemade basics like almond milk, almond yogurt, hummus, and protein pancakes.
- Simple, oil-free salad dressings.
- Practical notes on portion control, protein powders, hydration, turmeric use, and why certain foods (like flax and fruit-only juices) are excluded.

This section is not a substitute for medical or dietician guidance. It is my memoir in practice a clear, structured resource showing how food became a central tool in my healing and thriving.

Section 1: Juices

Juicing became the foundation of my mornings. Every juice is paired with protein because my oncology dieticians taught me never to take fruit-only juices. Fruit alone spikes blood sugar and leaves the gut empty too quickly, so I always balance with plant protein powder and sometimes psyllium husk for fiber.

Carrot Celery Kale Juice (Core Morning Juice)

Ingredients

- 3 medium carrots
- 2 celery stalks
- 1 cucumber
- 2 kale leaves
- ½ lemon, peeled
- 25 g vegan protein powder (pea, mung, or chickpea; single-ingredient only)
- (Optional) 1 tsp psyllium husk

Method

Wash all vegetables thoroughly.

Juice carrots, celery, cucumber, kale, and lemon.

Stir in protein powder until smooth.

Add psyllium husk if extra fiber is desired.

Drink immediately.

Health Note: Anti-inflammatory, rich in carotenoids, vitamin C, and alkalizing greens.

Beetroot Carrot Ginger Juice

Ingredients

- 1 small beetroot
- 2 medium carrots
- 1 cucumber
- 2 spinach leaves
- 1-inch fresh ginger
- ½ lemon
- 25 g vegan protein powder

Method

Juice beetroot, carrots, cucumber, spinach, ginger, and lemon.

Stir in protein powder.

Drink fresh.

Health Note: Excellent for blood health and boosting iron, especially valuable for cancer thrivers.

Kiwi Celery Spinach Juice

Ingredients

- 1 kiwi (peeled)
- 2 celery stalks
- 1 cucumber
- 2 spinach leaves
- 1-inch ginger
- 25 g vegan protein powder

Method

Juice celery, cucumber, spinach, kiwi, and ginger.

Mix in protein powder.

Drink right away.

Health Note: High in vitamin C, supports immunity, gentle on digestion.

Green Apple Kale Juice (Skin Only)

Ingredients

- Peel of ½ green apple (skin only)
- 2 kale leaves
- 2 celery stalks
- 1 cucumber
- 1-inch ginger
- 25 g vegan protein powder

Method

Juice apple peel, kale, celery, cucumber, and ginger.

Stir in protein powder.

Health Note: Provides polyphenols with reduced sugar.

Wheatgrass Juice (Started August 2021)

Ingredients

Fresh homegrown wheatgrass (a handful, ~30 ml juice yield)

Method

Plant wheatgrass in trays indoors using water only (no soil).

Allow grass to grow 6–8 inches.

Cut and juice immediately using a manual or electric wheatgrass juicer.

Drink first thing in the morning, on an empty stomach, before having any meal.

Drink immediately **NEVER store for later.**

Health Note: Rich in chlorophyll, which structurally resembles hemoglobin. Studies show wheatgrass can induce cancer cell death, reduce spread, and lower tumor formation in lab settings. Avoid supplements; fresh juice is safest.

Section 2: Smoothies

Smoothies were my evening meals light, healing, and balanced with leafy greens, a small cruciferous vegetable portion, a healthy fat, vegan protein powder, and fruit. Sometimes I added a small piece of ginger or fresh herbs for extra anti-inflammatory support. These smoothies were designed to be complete meals, not snacks.

Note on spinach: When using spinach in smoothies, I sometimes lightly steam it for 1–2 minutes before cooling and blending. This reduces oxalates, which can block calcium absorption, and makes antioxidants like lutein and beta-carotene more bioavailable. Light steaming does not destroy nutrients but helps the body use them better.

Blueberry Spinach Smoothie

Ingredients

- 1 cup unsweetened almond milk
- 1 cup spinach (lightly steamed & cooled before blending)
- ½ cup blueberries
- ¼ small avocado
- 25 g vegan protein powder (pea, mung, or chickpea)
- Small piece of fresh ginger

Method

Add all ingredients to a blender.

Blend until smooth.

Serve immediately.

Health Note: Antioxidant-rich, calcium-friendly, supports gut health.

Strawberry Kale Smoothie

Ingredients

- 1 cup unsweetened almond milk
- 1 kale leaf (small, de-stemmed)
- ½ cup strawberries
- 1 Tbsp hemp seeds
- 25 g vegan protein powder
- Pinch of cinnamon

Method

Combine all ingredients in blender.

Blend until creamy.

Serve fresh.

Health Note: Supports bone health, rich in vitamin C and omega-3s.

Raspberry Spinach Carrot Smoothie

Ingredients

- 1 cup unsweetened almond milk
- 1 cup spinach (lightly steamed & cooled)
- ½ cup raspberries
- 1 small carrot (peeled, chopped)
- 1 Tbsp chia seeds
- 25 g vegan protein powder

Method

Add all ingredients into blender.

Blend until smooth and creamy.

Serve immediately.

Health Note: Boosts beta-carotene, iron, and antioxidants.

Blackberry Arugula Smoothie

Ingredients

- 1 cup unsweetened almond milk
- 1 small handful arugula
- ½ cup blackberries
- 1 Tbsp chia seeds
- 25 g vegan protein powder
- Fresh mint or basil leaves (optional)

Method

Place all ingredients in blender.

Blend until smooth.

Drink right away.

Health Note: Peppery arugula adds cruciferous benefit; berries provide strong antioxidant support.

Cinnamon Broccoli Leaf Smoothie

Ingredients

- 1 cup unsweetened almond milk
- 1 small broccoli floret (lightly steamed & cooled)
- 1 cup spinach
- ½ green apple (skin only)
- 1 Tbsp hemp seeds
- 25 g vegan protein powder
- Pinch of cinnamon

Method

Blend all ingredients together until smooth.

Serve cold.

Health Note: Adds cruciferous protection in a gentle portion; cinnamon aids blood sugar balance.

Section 3: Soups

Soups were a cornerstone of my healing journey easy to digest, gentle on the gut, and nourishing with protein, fiber, and anti-inflammatory ingredients. Each recipe here balances vegetables with a protein base and avoids heavy starches, ensuring variety and cultural relevance.

Carrot Ginger Mung Bean Soup

Ingredients

- 2 medium carrots, peeled and chopped
- ½ cup cooked mung beans
- 1-inch fresh ginger
- 3 cups low-sodium vegetable broth
- Fresh parsley for garnish

Method

Simmer carrots, mung beans, ginger, and broth for 20 minutes.

Blend until smooth.

Serve warm, garnished with parsley.

Health Note: Light, soothing, and protein-rich with anti-inflammatory ginger.

Spinach Chickpea Soup

Ingredients

- 1 cup cooked chickpeas
- 2 cups spinach
- 1 small carrot (optional, for sweetness)
- 1 stalk celery, chopped
- 1 tsp turmeric + ½ tsp black pepper
- 3 cups vegetable broth (low sodium)

Method

Combine chickpeas, spinach, carrot, celery, turmeric, and broth in a pot.

Simmer for 20 minutes until vegetables are soft.

Blend half the soup for creaminess and leave the rest chunky.

Serve warm.

Health Note: Leafy greens with protein; turmeric and black pepper enhance anti-inflammatory effect.

Zucchini Green Pea Soup

Ingredients

- 1 medium zucchini, chopped
- 1 cup green peas
- 1 small onion, chopped
- 1 clove garlic (optional, if tolerated)
- 3 cups vegetable broth (low sodium)
- Fresh basil leaves

Method

In a pot, simmer zucchini, peas, onion, garlic, and broth for 20 minutes.

Blend until smooth.

Add basil before serving.

Health Note: IBS-friendly, creamy texture with plant protein and antioxidants.

Butternut–Cannellini Bean Soup

Ingredients

- ½ cup butternut squash, cubed
- 1 cup cannellini beans (cooked)
- ½ cup unsweetened almond milk
- 1-inch ginger
- 3 cups vegetable broth (low sodium)
- Fresh coriander for garnish

Method

Combine butternut, beans, ginger, and broth in a pot.

Simmer 20 minutes until tender.

Blend until smooth and stir in almond milk.

Serve with fresh coriander.

Health Note: Balanced with small starch (butternut), protein (beans), and creaminess from almond milk.

Omena Vegetable Soup

Ingredients

- 120 g omena (anchovies), soaked and cleaned
- 1 medium tomato, chopped
- 1 small onion, chopped
- 1 cup spinach or kale
- 3 cups vegetable broth (low sodium)
- Fresh coriander or parsley for garnish

Method

Soak omena in warm water for 15 minutes.

Simmer omena, tomato, onion, and broth for 20 minutes.

Add spinach/kale in the last 5 minutes.

Serve warm with herbs.

Health Note: High in protein and calcium; perfect for bone health and cultural balance.

Section 5: Salad Dressings

Salads became my go-to lunch during treatment and beyond. They were quick to pack, nutritionally complete with beans or legumes, and reduced stress during workdays. These simple, oil-free dressings kept each salad flavorful, anti-inflammatory, and clean.

Citrus Herb Dressing

Ingredients

- ¼ cup fresh orange juice
- 2 Tbsp lemon juice
- 1 Tbsp chia seeds
- 2 Tbsp chopped parsley or cilantro

Method

Whisk all ingredients together in a small bowl.

Let sit 5–10 minutes for chia to thicken.

Health Note: Bright, refreshing; chia adds fiber and healthy omega-3s.

Avocado Lime Ranch (Cleaned-Up)

Ingredients

- ¼ small avocado
- 3 Tbsp lime juice
- 2 Tbsp almond milk (unsweetened)
- 1 Tbsp fresh dill
- 1 Tbsp chopped parsley

Method

Mash avocado until smooth.

Whisk in lime juice, almond milk, dill, and parsley until creamy.

Health Note: Creamy and oil-free; avocado provides healthy fats without heaviness.

Ginger Turmeric Dressing

Ingredients

- 1 tsp grated fresh ginger
- ½ tsp ground turmeric
- 2 Tbsp lemon juice
- Pinch black pepper
- 1 Tbsp chopped basil

Method

Whisk ginger, turmeric, lemon juice, and black pepper together.

Stir in fresh basil before serving.

Health Note: Anti-inflammatory powerhouse; black pepper enhances turmeric absorption.

Berry Mint Dressing

Ingredients

- ¼ cup raspberries or blueberries (pureed)
- 1 Tbsp chopped mint leaves
- 1 Tbsp rice vinegar

Method

Blend berries into a smooth puree.

Whisk in mint and rice vinegar.

Health Note: Sweet-tart option; rich in antioxidants, pairs well with legumes.

Classic Lemon Chia Dressing

Ingredients

- 3 Tbsp fresh lemon juice
- 2 Tbsp water
- 1 Tbsp chia seeds
- 1 Tbsp chopped parsley or cilantro

Method

Whisk all ingredients together.

Allow to sit for 5 minutes for chia to swell and thicken.

Health Note: Simple, light, and protein-friendly; boosts hydration and omega-3s.

Section 6: Special Notes and Guidance

This section brings together the key lessons I learned from oncology nutritionists, dieticians, and my own journey. It is not medical advice but a practical guide for anyone navigating cancer treatment, recovery, or simply looking for a clean, healing diet. Each note is explained in detail to turn every stone for those seeking clarity.

Hydration

I aim for close to a gallon of water each day about 7 bottles of 500 ml. Hydration is essential for digestion, cellular repair, joint health, and detoxification. Dehydration during chemotherapy or radiation can worsen fatigue, nausea, and constipation. Warm water with a pinch of Himalayan salt and lemon, taken 30 minutes before workouts, prepared my body for exercise by replenishing electrolytes and waking up my metabolism.

Protein Powders

Protein was central to my healing. It helped preserve muscle mass, repair tissues, and keep my weight in a safe range. Oncology dieticians emphasized one strict rule: only use vegan powders with a single ingredient — such as pea, mung bean, or chickpea protein. Powders with long lists of additives, sugars, or artificial flavors are not safe for thrivers. I personally read labels carefully; if I don't recognize an ingredient, I don't use it.

Protein Powder Brands that I Use:
- Naked Pea Protein — 100% yellow pea protein, no additives.
- Solo Organic Pea Protein Isolate - , Low in Sodium, 100% Vegan, Non-GMO, Unflavored Plant Based Protein Powder. Keto & Paleo Friendly, No Additives
- Anthony's Premium Pea Protein — affordable, clean, widely used.
- Terrasoul Superfood Protein Powders — single-ingredient, sprouted option.
- Growing Naturals Raw Pea Protein Powder, Vegan Plant Based Protein, BCAA, Low-Carb, Low-Sugar, Original Unflavored
- Based Classic Sprouted Brown Rice Protein Powder Natural by Sunwarrior

Turmeric

Turmeric in cooking is safe and beneficial. Curcumin, its active compound, has anti-inflammatory and antioxidant properties. When combined with black pepper, absorption improves significantly. I use turmeric freely in cooking, paired with pepper for best results.

However, turmeric supplements are not recommended for breast cancer thrivers. Supplements deliver extremely high doses of curcumin, which can interfere with cancer medications (like estrogen inhibitors and some chemotherapy drugs). The supplement market is poorly regulated, making it impossible to guarantee purity. Other risks include blood thinning (increasing surgical risk) and digestive irritation (bloating, nausea, reflux).

My oncologist and nutrition team were very clear: spices in food are healing, supplements are risky. Safety comes from consuming turmeric as part of a balanced diet, not as a concentrated pill.

Oils in Cooking and Charred Foods

I rarely use oils in my own diet. My healthy fats come from avocado slices, chia seeds, and hemp seeds, whole and natural. However, for my family, I occasionally use three oils recommended by my oncology dieticians. Each has a different smoking point — the temperature at which oil begins to break down and produce harmful compounds:

- Olive Oil: Smoking point - 375°F (190°C). Best for salads or very low heat cooking.
- Avocado Oil: Smoking point - 520°F (270°C). Safest for high heat cooking like sautéing, baking, or frying eggs.
- Canola Oil: Smoking point - 400°F (204°C). Acceptable for moderate heat; rarely used.

Smoking point matters because when oils are heated past their limit, they release toxic compounds like acrylamide, polycyclic aromatic hydrocarbons (PAHs), and advanced glycation end products (AGEs). These are linked to inflammation, oxidative stress, and higher risk of cancer.

Charred foods are equally dangerous. The blackened parts of roasted corn, barbecued meats, or even over-crisped vegetables contain carcinogens such as PAHs and heterocyclic amines (HCAs). These form when fats and juices drip onto flames or when food is cooked directly over high heat.

Examples of risky foods if charred:

- Nyama choma (grilled meat)
- Roasted corn with blackened kernels
- Burnt chapati or vegetables
- Over-crisped chicken skin

Safer practices include steaming, boiling, air frying, or baking at moderate temperatures. If roasting, wrap foods to avoid direct burning, and always trim away any blackened portions before eating. For my own meals, I strictly avoid roasting to eliminate the risk altogether.

Personalized Portion Control

Dieticians used my BMI to calculate my daily needs for protein, fiber, and calories. Every cancer thriver is different. It is dangerous to copy another person's plate. For those without access to a dietician, a simple hand guide works.

- Protein = palm of your hand
- Carbohydrates = cupped hand (minimal)
- Vegetables = two open hands
- Fats = thumb

During chemotherapy, I ate three meals and two snacks (I also drank a midnight shake to cushion my gut). After treatment, I reduced it to two meals and a juice breakfast, as my energy and schedule changed.

Figure 3.1: Serving Size Guide by MD Anderson

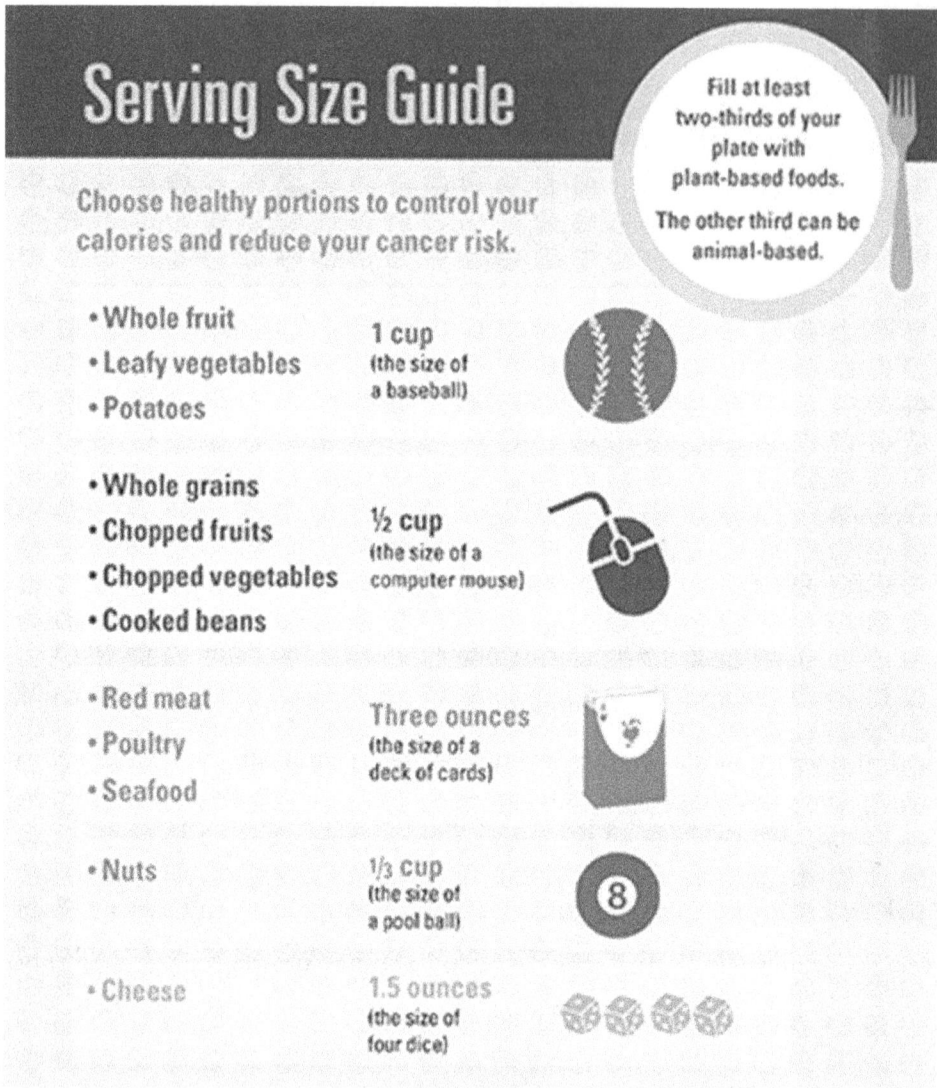

Serving Size Guide

Fill at least two-thirds of your plate with plant-based foods.

The other third can be animal-based.

Choose healthy portions to control your calories and reduce your cancer risk.

- Whole fruit
- Leafy vegetables
- Potatoes

1 cup (the size of a baseball)

- Whole grains
- Chopped fruits
- Chopped vegetables
- Cooked beans

½ cup (the size of a computer mouse)

- Red meat
- Poultry
- Seafood

Three ounces (the size of a deck of cards)

- Nuts

⅓ cup (the size of a pool ball)

- Cheese

1.5 ounces (the size of four dice)

Source: Adapted from The University of Texas MD Anderson Cancer Center – Healthy Eating Plate and Portion Guide.

Supplements

The only supplements I take, with my oncologist's approval, are calcium, vitamin D, and multivitamins. Other supplements marketed for cancer are unsafe because of poor regulation and possible drug interactions.

Some Recommended Clean Brands:
- Calcium: Citracal Slow Release, Nature Made Calcium Citrate.
- Vitamin D: Pure Encapsulations Vitamin D3, Thorne Vitamin D/K2.
- Multivitamin: Pure Encapsulations O.N.E. Multivitamin, Garden of Life mykind Organics Women's Multi.

Calcium is essential because estrogen inhibitors (like anastrozole, exemestane) reduce bone density. Vitamin D supports breast and bone health, while multivitamin helps fill small gaps when appetite or diet is limited. I only use pure encapsulated or certified clean brands.

PART FOUR

The Cheat Page

This final chapter is a practical tool for cancer patients and caregivers. It contains the key questions you need to ask your doctors, the reasoning behind some of my own major decisions, and an explanation of critical medical terms that are often misunderstood.

Key Questions Every Patient Should Ask Their Doctor

1. What is my prognosis?

Ask directly about your chances and treatment options. Prognosis helps you plan realistically.

2. What receptors does the tumor have?

Insist on knowing if it is estrogen receptor-positive, progesterone receptor-positive, HER2, or triple negative.

3. After surgery, are my margins clear?

Ask how far the tumor was from the margin and whether cancer cells were completely removed.

Why I Made My Decisions

Double/Bilateral Mastectomy

I chose this path because I did not want to live with the constant anxiety of repeated breast scans. Flat closure gave me peace and allowed me to feel my chest wall clearly and without worry about cancer moving from one breast to another.

Total Hysterectomy (Ovaries + Uterus Removed): The tumor had estrogen receptors, and I did not want to give hormonal cancers another chance. Even though estrogen inhibitors suppress hormones, ovaries can begin producing them again after treatment stops. Removing my ovaries and uterus was, for me, an extra layer of protection against this specific tumor. I did not make this decision to prevent all other types of cancers. I am also aware that even with this precaution, the cancer tumor may still recur.

Understanding the Terms: Remission, Survivor, NED, Cancer-Free

Remission: This begins immediately after treatment when scans show no visible cancer. It means the cancer is controlled, but monitoring is still required.

Survivor: At MD Anderson and many hospitals, patients are considered survivors after reaching the 5-year mark without recurrence. At this point, many are moved from active oncology to survivorship programs.

No Evidence of Disease (NED): NED is not declared right after treatment. It usually comes years later, after repeated scans and bloodwork consistently show no return of cancer. It reflects stability and time-tested healing.

Cancer-Free: Doctors generally avoid this term because medicine cannot guarantee that cancer will never return. However, some oncologists may cautiously use 'cancer free' to describe the original primary cancer site if a patient has been in long-term NED and the risk of that cancer returning is extremely low. This is not a guarantee against new cancers developing, but it does recognize that the original cancer is no longer active after years of surveillance.

Why this matters: Doctors should never say 'cancer-free' immediately after treatment. It can be misleading and emotionally harmful if recurrence happens. The truthful path is remission → survivor → NED → and for some, eventually hearing 'cancer free' from their oncologist in relation to the original cancer.

Final Empowering Note

Every patient's journey is unique. What I chose worked for me, but it may not be the same for you. The key is to ask questions boldly, listen to your body, and make decisions that bring you peace. Do not be rushed. Knowledge, honesty, and clarity are part of healing.

Reader's Notes

Take a few moments to reflect and personalize your journey. Use the pages that follow to set goals, track meals, or simply write what nourishes your soul.

My 3 health goals after reading *Nourished to Thrive* are:

1. _____

2. _____

3. _____

Foods that make me feel energized:

_____

_____

Habit I want to build or strengthen:

_____

_____

Remember: healing happens in small, consistent steps. Your body listens when you care for it.

Dedication to Cancer Thrivers

This book is lovingly dedicated to every cancer warrior, survivor, and thriver — those still fighting, those in remission, and those who loved themselves enough to keep trying.

May your story remind the world that cancer may touch your body, but it cannot touch your will to live, your faith, or your joy. You are not merely surviving — you are thriving!

About the Author

Dr. Diana C. Awuor, Ed.D. is a Fulbright Scholar, U.S. Presidential Lifetime Achievement Award Honoree, and breast cancer thriver who turned her pain into purpose. Diagnosed with breast cancer in 2020 while caring for a newborn and pursuing her doctorate, she chose faith, discipline, and nutrition as her path to healing.

She is the Founder and Executive Director of International Pleroma Convocation, an organizations dedicated to promoting cancer awareness, early detection, and nutritional healing.

A university educator, author, and international public speaker, Dr. Awuor uses her platform to mentor, educate, and empower others to live full and purposeful lives. Her mission is simple yet profound: to help others thrive through nourishment — of body, mind, and spirit.

Connect with Dr. Diana Awuor

To stay inspired and connected:

Instagram: @CandidDiana

Website: www.dianawuor.com

Email: contact@dianawuor.com

TikTok: @CandidDiana

Follow the conversation and share your journey using the hashtag **#NourishedToThrive**.

Dr. Awuor loves hearing from readers — your stories, recipes, and testimonies may inspire others on their own path to healing.

Invite Dr. Diana to Speak

Dr. Diana Awuor is a renowned International Public Speaker who delivers transformative talks on Cancer Awareness, Hope, Healing, and Life After Cancer. She also facilitates the inspiring Pain to Purpose Workshop — a faith-based mentoring experience that helps individuals find meaning, resilience, and renewed purpose after trauma.

Invite Dr. Diana to your church, conference, corporate event, or wellness retreat to empower your audience with a message of strength, courage, and holistic living.

Website: www.dianawuor.com
Email: contact@dianawuor.com

"Her story is a testimony that faith and nourishment can rebuild what pain once destroyed."

Other Books by Dr. Diana C. Awuor

Faith & Healing Titles

- Pain to Purpose Devotional: A 5-Day Journey of Healing, Faith, and Hope

- Ensnared: The Toxicity of Anger, Delayed Forgiveness, and Prolonged Grudges

Available on Amazon and through Candid Diana Press.

"You can heal and still live a beautiful life."

Every time you choose whole foods, gratitude, and self-kindness, you tell your body that it deserves love. May you continue to nourish yourself with wisdom, courage, and peace — and may your healing inspire others to do the same.

With love,

Dr. Diana C. Awuor

www.ingramcontent.com/pod-product-compliance
Lightning Source LLC
Chambersburg PA
CBHW080555270326
41929CB00019B/3321